# The Theology of Medicine

W9-BJJ-264

*Other books by Thomas Szasz*

Pain and Pleasure
The Myth of Mental Illness
Law, Liberty, and Psychiatry
Psychiatric Justice
The Ethics of Psychoanalysis
The Manufacture of Madness
Ideology and Insanity
The Age of Madness (Ed.)
The Second Sin
Ceremonial Chemistry
Heresies
Karl Kraus and the Soul-Doctors
Schizophrenia
Psychiatric Slavery
The Myth of Psychotherapy
Sex by Prescription
The Therapeutic State
Insanity

# The Theology of Medicine

## THE POLITICAL-PHILOSOPHICAL FOUNDATIONS OF MEDICAL ETHICS

*Thomas Szasz*

SYRACUSE UNIVERSITY PRESS

Copyright © 1977, 1988 by Thomas Szasz

*All Rights Reserved*

Syracuse University Press Edition 1988
93 92 91 90 89 88 6 5 4 3 2 1

The paper used in this publication meets the minimum requirements of American National Standard for Information Sciences—Permanence of Paper for Printed Library Materials, ANSI Z39.48-1984. ∞™

**Library of Congress Cataloging-in-Publication Data**

Szasz, Thomas Stephen, 1920–
The theology of medicine : the poltiical-philosphical foundations of medical ethics / Thomas Szasz.
p. cm.
Reprint. Originally published: Ne wYork : Harper & Row, 1977.
Includes bibliographical references and index.
ISBN 0-8156-0225-1 (alk. paper)
1. Medical ethics. 2. Psychiatric ethics. I. Title.
[DNLM: 1. Ethics, Medical—history—collected works.
2. Philosophy, Medical—collected works. 3. Politics—collected works. 4. Religion and Medicine—collected works. W 50 S996t 1977a]
R724.S97 1988
174'.2—dc19
DNLM/DLC
for Library of Congress 87-26769
CIP

Manufactured in the United States of America

Had not the Roman government permitted free inquiry, Christianity could never have been introduced. Had not free inquiry been indulged at the era of the Reformation, the corruptions of Christianity could not have been purged away. If it be restrained now, the present corruptions will be protected, and new ones encouraged. Was the government to prescribe to us our medicine and diet, our bodies would be in such keeping as our souls are now.

Thomas Jefferson, "Notes on the State of Virginia" (1781)

# Contents

# Preface

The essays assembled in this volume reflect my long-standing interest in moral philosophy and my conviction that the idea of a medical ethics as something distinct and separate from ethics is an absurdity. Every person who *acts* is a *moral agent*. A person who possesses special knowledge and skills and is expected to act in the face of life-threatening circumstances—such as a physician—is someone whose status as moral agent is accordingly greatly enhanced. By this I simply mean that the moral character of medical actions is, in general, more intense than that of ordinary, everyday human actions. Perhaps because this fact presents us with so many vexing moral dilemmas, there has developed an almost contrary view, namely, that the physician acts in a sort of moral vacuum—on a morally elevated plane, to be sure—but in a vacuum, nonetheless, in which the only concern is the health of the patient. This is a dangerous piece of nonsense, its nonsensical character more painfully evident every day.

The quintessentially moral character of medicine has, of course, been recognized since ancient times, when, indeed, the distinctions among medical healing, moral philosophy, and religion were vague or nonexistent. As these distinctions developed, problems of medical ethics began to surface. Such problems play a prominent role in the works of numerous philosophers, playwrights, and novelists. Plato, Shakespeare, Molière, Ibsen, Shaw, among those who easily come to mind, have all addressed issues we would now classify as medico-ethical. Perhaps less well known is one of Karel Capek's plays, *Power and Glory*, which is devoted entirely to the problem of the relations among medicine, ethics, and politics. The scenario, briefly, is as follows.

A world-wide epidemic erupts. The disease affects only older persons, "everyone round about fifty catches it sooner or later."* In an early

*Capek, K., *Power and Glory: A Drama in Three Acts*, English version by Paul Selver and Ralph Neale (London: George Allen & Unwin, 1938), p. 28.

scene, a father, worried about catching the disease, wonders aloud to his family, "But why at that age? Why?" His daughter replies: "To give the younger ones a chance to make a living, I suppose. There're so many old people living nowadays that we've hardly elbow room" (p. 28).

Professor Sigelius, a representative of the establishment, stands helpless in the face of the epidemic. At the same time, we learn that Dr. Galen, an obscure physician, has a cure for the disease but is willing to treat only poor and unimportant patients. Sought out by eager journalists, Galen explains his position: "If men go on murdering each other with bullets and poison gas, why should doctors be expected to try and save them from any other death? . . . If the powerful and the rich really want peace, it is theirs for the asking" (p. 46–47).

Professor Sigelius interrupts him, telling the reporters: "He's very near to a nervous breakdown. You'll please forget anything he may have said to you!" (p. 47). After the journalists leave, Sigelius confronts Galen:

> PROFESSOR. You're either crazy or you're determined to be arrested on a charge of treason. Don't you realize the political situation?
>
> GALEN. I do.
>
> PROFESSOR. Well, you're a doctor. It's your duty to cure the sick. That's all you have to think of [p. 48].

Galen tries to explain himself, but Sigelius dismisses him: "I'm not merely a doctor. I'm a servant of my country. Good-bye Dr. Galen" (p. 49). As the play ends, with the nation at the brink of war, Galen is trampled to death by a patriotically intoxicated mob.

Capek dramatizes the central problem of medical ethics, namely: Whose agent is the physician? Surely, this question and the implications of the true answer to it are no less momentous today than they were a half a century ago.

Syracuse, New York
September 1987

Thomas Szasz

# Preface to First Edition

This book is a collection of essays most of which have appeared previously. Many of them, however, were first prepared for lectures and were subsequently published in a shorter version than the original text from which they were excerpted. I have retained the full-length versions of these essays and some of them—for example, "The Ethics of Addiction" and "The Ethics of Suicide"—are published in this form here for the first time.

I thank the editors and publishers of the journals and books in which these pieces first appeared for granting permission for their republication; Cynthia Merman of Harper & Row for help with the selection and editing of the essays for publication in book form; and Debbie Murphy, my secretary, for her customarily devoted labors.

# Acknowledgments

Grateful acknowledgment is made to the following sources for permission to use the articles that appear in this volume in adapted form:

"The Moral Physician." Adapted from "The Moral Physician," *The Center Magazine,* vol. 8 (March–April 1975), pp. 2–9.

"Illness and Indignity." Adapted from "Illness and Indignity," *The Journal of the American Medical Association*, vol. 227 (February 1974), pp. 543–545. Copyright 1974, American Medical Association. Reprinted by permission.

"The Ethics of Addiction." Adapted from "The Ethics of Addiction," *Harper's Magazine*, April 1972, pp. 74–79.

"The Ethics of Suicide." Adapted from "The Ethics of Suicide," *The Antioch Review*, vol. 31 (Spring 1971), pp. 7–17.

"Language and Lunacy." Adapted from "Language and Humanism." This article first appeared in *The Humanist*, January/February 1974, and is reprinted by permission.

"The Right to Health." Adapted from "The Right to Health," *The Georgetown Law Journal*, vol. 57 (March 1969), pp. 734–751. Reprinted by permission.

"Justice in the Therapeutic State." Adapted from "Justice in the Therapeutic State," in *The Administration of Justice in America: The 1968–69 E. Paul du Pont Lectures on Crime, Delinquency, and Corrections* (Newark, Del.: University of Delaware Press, 1970), pp. 75–92.

"The Illogic and Immorality of Involuntary Psychiatric Interventions: A Personal Restatement." Adapted from "The Danger of

Coercive Psychiatry," *American Bar Association Journal*, vol. 61 (October 1975), pp. 1246–1249.

"The Metaphors of Faith and Folly." Adapted from "Medical Metaphorology," *American Psychologist*, vol. 30 (August 1975), pp. 859–861. Copyright 1975 by the American Psychological Association. Reprinted by permission.

"Medicine and the State: A *Humanist* Interview." Adapted from "Medicine and the State: The First Amendment Violated—An Interview with Thomas Szasz." This article first appeared in *The Humanist*, March/April 1973, and is reprinted by permission.

# Introduction

The crucial moral characteristic of the human condition is the dual experience of freedom of the will and personal responsibility. Since freedom and responsibility are two aspects of the same phenomenon, they invite comparison with the proverbial knife that cuts both ways. One of its edges implies options: we call it freedom. The other implies obligations: we call it responsibility. People like freedom because it gives them mastery over things and people. They dislike responsibility because it constrains them from satisfying their wants. That is why one of the things that characterizes history is the unceasing human effort to maximize freedom and minimize responsibility. But to no avail, for each real increase in human freedom —whether in the Garden of Eden or in the Nevada desert, in the chemical laboratory or in the medical laboratory—brings with it a proportionate increase in responsibility. Each exhilaration with the power to do good is soon eclipsed by the guilt for having used it to do evil.

Confronted with this inexorable fact of life, human beings have sought to bend it to their own advantage, or at least to what they thought was their advantage. In the main, people have done so by ascribing their freedom, and hence also their responsibility, to some agency outside themselves. They have thus projected their own moral qualities onto others—moralizing them and demoralizing themselves. In the process, they have made others into puppeteers and themselves into puppets.

Evidently, the oldest scheme for constructing such an arrangement is religion: only deities have free will and responsibility; people are mere puppets. Although most religions temper this imagery by attributing some measure of self-action to the puppets, the importance of the underlying world view can hardly be exaggerated. Indeed, people still often try to explain the behavior of certain self-sacrificing persons by saying that they are carrying out God's will; and, perhaps more important still, people often claim to be carrying out God's will when they sacrifice others, whether in a religious crusade or in a so-called psychotic episode. The important thing about this imagery is that it makes us witness to, and even participants in, a human drama in which the actors are seen as robots, their movements being directed by unseen, and indeed invisible, higher powers.

If stated so simply and starkly, many people nowadays might be inclined to dismiss this imagery as something only a religious fanatic would entertain. That would be a grave mistake, as it would blind us to the fact that it is precisely this imagery that animates much contemporary religious, political, medical, psychiatric, and scientific thought. How else are we to account for the systematic invocation of divinities by national leaders? Or the use of the Bible, the Talmud, the Koran, or other holy books as guides to the proper channeling of one's freedom to act in the world? One of the universal solvents for guilt, engendered by the undesirable consequences of one's actions, is God. That is why religion used to be, and still is, an important social institution.

But the belief in deities as puppeteers and in people as puppets has diminished during the past few centuries. There has, however, been no corresponding increase in the human acceptance of, and tolerance for, personal responsibility and individual guilt. People still try to convince themselves that they are not responsible, or are responsible only to a very limited extent, for the undesirable consequences of their behavior. How else are we to account for the systematic invocation of Marx and Mao by national leaders? Or the use of the writings of Freud, Spock, and other ostensibly scientific works as guides to the proper channeling of one's freedom to act in the world? Today, the universal solvent for guilt is science. That is why medicine is such an important social institution.

For millennia, men and women escaped from responsibility by theologizing morals. Now they escape from it by medicalizing morals. Then, if God approved a particular conduct, it was good; and if He disapproved it, it was bad. How did people know what God approved and disapproved? The Bible—that is to say, the biblical experts, called priests—told them so. Today, if Medicine approves a particular conduct, it is good; and if it disapproves it, it is bad. And how do people know what Medicine approves or disapproves? Medicine—that is to say, the medical experts, called physicians—tells them so.

The extermination of heretics in Christian pyres was a theological matter. The extermination of Jews in Nazi gas chambers was a medical matter. The inquisitorial destruction of the traditional legal procedures of Continental courts was a theological matter. The psychiatric destruction of the rule of law in American courts is a medical matter. And so it goes.

Human life—that is, a life of consciousness and self-awareness—is unimaginable without suffering. Without pain and sorrow, there could be no pleasure and joy; just as without death, there could be no life; without illness, no health; without ugliness, no beauty; without poverty, no riches; and so on ad infinitum with the countless human experiences we categorize as undesirable and desirable.

All our exertions—moral and medical, political and personal—are directed toward minimizing undesirable experiences and maximizing desirable ones. However, if the calculus of personal conduct could be reduced to such a simple prudential principle, human life would be much less complicated than it is. What complicates it of course is the fact that many of the things we regard as desirable are opposed by, or can be secured only at the cost of, others that we regard as also desirable. There seems to be no limit to the internal conflicts and contradictions among the things we abstractly value and wish to maximize. For example, enjoyable eating or drinking often conflicts with good health, sexual pleasure often conflicts with dignity, liberty often conflicts with security, and so on. This is, quite simply, why the pursuit of relief from suffering, reasonable though it may seem, cannot be an unqualified personal or political goal. And if we make it such a goal, it is certain to result in more, not less, suffering. In the past, the greatest unhappiness for the greatest number was thus created by precisely those political programs whose goal was the most radical relief of suffering for the greatest number of human beings. While those campaigns against suffering were in progress, people viewed them with unqualified approval; now we look back at them as the most terrifying tyrannies.

In the absence of the perfect vision that comes only with hindsight, let us at least try to look at our own age critically. If we do so we shall glimpse—or even see clearly enough—the contours of two contemporary ideologies that have set themselves this same perennial goal—namely, the radical relief of suffering for the greatest numbers. One of these, holding the East in its grip, is the Marxist-Communist campaign against unhappiness: it promises total relief from suffering through victory over capitalism, the ultimate cause of all human misery. The other, holding the West in its grip, is the scientific-medical campaign against unhappiness: it promises total relief from suffering through victory over disease, the ultimate cause of all human misery.

In countries under Communist rule, where its efforts to relieve suffering are unchecked by any effective countervailing force, Communism has thus succeeded in being the greatest source of suffering; whereas in the so-called free West, where "therapeutism" has achieved a power unchecked by any effective countervailing force, Medicine has succeeded in becoming one of the greatest sources of suffering.

How medicine, the art of healing, has changed from man's ally into his adversary, and how it has done so during the very decades when its powers to heal have advanced the most momentously during its whole history—that is a story whose telling must await another occasion, perhaps even another narrator. It must suffice here to note that there is nothing new about the fact that in human affairs the power to do good is usually commensurate with, if not exceeded by, the power to do evil; that human ingenuity has created, especially in the institutions of Anglo-American law and politics, arrangements that have proved useful in dividing the power to do good into its two basic components—namely, *good* and *power*; and that these institutional arrangements, and the moral principles they embody, have sought to promote the good by depriving its producers and purveyors of power over those desiring to receive or reject their services. The most outstanding monument to that effort on the part of rulers to protect their subjects from those who would do them good, even if it meant doing them in, is the First Amendment clause guaranteeing that "Congress shall make no law respecting an establishment of religion, or prohibiting the free exercise thereof." Let me indicate briefly how I think that guaranty, and the moral and political principles it embodies, applies to our contemporary conditions.

Everyone now recognizes the reality of spiritual suffering—that is, of the fact that men, women, and children may be, and often are, distressed because they can neither find nor give meaning to their lives, or because they can neither accept nor create satisfactory standards for regulating their personal conduct. Although these circumstances result in untold suffering, no one in the United States—certainly, no judicial or legal authorities—would contend that such unhappiness justifies the forcible imposition of certain religious beliefs and practices on the sufferers. Such an intervention, even if it proved "helpful" in relieving the suffering, would violate the First Amendment guaranty against the "establishment of religion."

In the essays assembled in this volume, I try to show that this principle applies, and ought to be applied, to medical or so-called therapeutic interventions as well. I maintain, in other words, that suffering caused by illness—regardless of whether it is actual bodily illness or alleged mental illness—cannot be the ground, in American law, for depriving a person of liberty, even if the incarceration is called *hospitalization*, and even if the intervention is called *treatment*. I contend that such use of state power—whether rationalized as the necessary deployment of the police power or as the therapeutic application of the principle of *parens patriae*—is contrary to the ideas and ideals enshrined in the First Amendment to the Constitution.

To join this argument, we need not consider what the state might do, or ought to do, *to* citizens who are *not* suffering in order to do something *for* those who *are*. The recipients of social security or welfare payments are not subjected to the police power of the state: they are not incarcerated and are not compelled to submit to medical treatments. However, we must consider what is being done in the United States—and, of course, elsewhere too—to people who are suffering, or who are alleged to be suffering, ostensibly to help them. It is precisely at this point that the theology of medicine—and especially the theology of psychiatry and of therapy—is writ clear and large.

For example, on February 6, 1976, *Psychiatric News*, the official newspaper of the American Psychiatric Association, published a front-page interview conducted by Robert Pear of the *Washington Star* with Dr. Judd Marmor, the president of the American Psychiatric Association. After alluding to my objections to involuntary psychiatric interventions, Pear asks Marmor, "But if a person who is supposedly ill doesn't recognize his illness and doesn't request treatment—should society intervene?" To which Marmor replies, "Yes, because these individuals are suffering and it's in the nature of their suffering very often that they are in no position to evaluate the fact that they are mentally ill."[1]

This modern therapeutic view seems to me identical to the traditional theological view according to which some persons are suffering and it's in the nature of their suffering very often that they are in no position to evaluate the fact that they have strayed from the true faith.

The framers of the Constitution opposed such sophistry and such policy. They reasoned—I think rightly—that even if the case were exactly as Marmor, for example, presents it, it should be enough for those solicitous for the welfare of such "sufferers" to offer them their "help." That would remove the sufferers' supposed ignorance about their own suffering and about the help available for its relief. Neither the existence of such suffering, real or alleged, nor the existence of help for it, real or alleged, could justify, in this view, an alliance between church and state and the use of the state's power to impose clerical help on unwilling clients. Just so, I insist, it cannot justify imposing clinical help on them.

How, then, has it come about that medicine has succeeded where religion has failed? How has therapy been able to breach the wall separating church and state where theology has been unable to do so? Briefly put, medicine has been able to achieve what religion has not, primarily by a radical violation of our vocabulary, of our conceptual categories; and secondarily, through the subversion of our ideals and institutions devoted to protecting us from reposing power in those who would help us whether we like it or not. We have done it before

1. "Marmor Hits Szasz for 'Enormous Distortions,'" *Psychiatric News*, February 6, 1976, p. 1.

to the blacks. Now we are doing it to each other, regardless of creed, color, or race.

How was slavery justified and made possible? By calling blacks *chattel* rather than *persons*. If blacks had been recognized as persons, there could have been no selling and buying of slaves, no fugitive slave laws—in short, there could have been no American slavery. And if plantations could be called *farms*, and forcing blacks to work on them could be called guaranteeing them their *right to work*, then slavery might still be regarded as compatible with the Constitution.[2] As it is, no term can now conceal that slavery is involuntary servitude. Nothing can. Whereas anything can now conceal the fact that institutional psychiatry is involuntary servitude.

How are involuntary psychiatric interventions—and the many other medical violations of individual freedom—justified and made possible? By calling people *patients*, imprisonment *hospitalization*, and torture *therapy*; and by calling uncomplaining individuals *sufferers*, medical and mental-health personnel who infringe on their liberty and dignity *therapists*, and the things the latter do to the former *treatments*. This is why such terms as *mental health* and the *right to treatment* now so effectively conceal that psychiatry is involuntary servitude.

It is at our own peril that we forget that language is our most important possession or tool; and that whereas in the language of science we explain events, in the language of morals we justify actions. We may thus explain abortion as a certain type of medical procedure but must justify permitting or prohibiting it by calling it *treatment* or the *murder of the unborn child*.

In everyday life, the distinction between explanation and justification is often blurred, and for a good reason. It is often difficult to know what one should do, what is a valid justification for engaging in a particular action. One of the best ways of resolving such uncertainty is to justify a particular course of action by claiming to explain it. We then say we have had no choice but to obey the Truth —as revealed by God or Science.

2. In this connection, see generally my *The Second Sin* (Garden City, N.Y.: Doubleday, Anchor Press, 1973) and *Heresies* (Garden City, N.Y.: Doubleday, Anchor Press, 1976).

Another reason for concealing justifications as explanations is that, rhetorically, a justification offered as such is often weak, whereas a justification put forth as an explanation is often very powerful. For example, formerly, if a man had justified his not eating by saying that he wanted to starve himself to death, he would have been considered mad; but if he had explained it by saying that he was doing so the better to serve God, he would have been regarded as devoutly religious. Similarly, today, if a slender woman justifies her not eating by saying she wants to lose weight, she is considered to be a madwoman suffering from anorexia nervosa; but if she explains it by saying that she is doing so to combat some political wrongdoing in the world, she is regarded as a noble protester against injustice.

To be sure, people do suffer. And that fact—according to doctors and patients, lawyers and laymen—is now enough to justify calling and considering them patients. As in an earlier age through the universality of sin, so now through the universality of suffering, men, women, and children become—whether they like it or not, whether they want to or not—the patient-penitents of their physician-priests. And over both patient and doctor now stands the Church of Medicine, its theology defining their roles and the rules of the games they must play, and its canon laws, now called *public health* and *mental health* laws, enforcing conformity to the dominant medical ethic.

My views on medical ethics depend heavily on the analogy between religion and medicine—between our freedom, or the lack of it, to accept or reject theological and therapeutic intervention. It seems obvious that in proportion as people value religion more highly than liberty, they will seek to ally religion with the state and support state-coerced theological practices; similarly, in proportion as they value medicine more highly than liberty, they will seek to ally medicine with the state and support state-coerced therapeutic practices. The point, simple but inexorable, is that when religion and liberty conflict, people must choose between theology and freedom; and that when medicine and liberty conflict, they must choose between therapy and freedom.

If Americans were confronted with this choice today, and if they regarded religion as highly as they regard medicine, they would no doubt try to reconcile what are irreconcilable—by calling incarceration in ecclesiastical institutions *the right to attend church* and torture on the rack *the right to practice the rituals of one's faith.* If the latter terms were accepted as the proper names of the former practices, coerced religious observance and religious persecution could be held to be constitutional. Those subjected to such practices could then be categorized as persons *guaranteed their right to religion*, and those who object to such violations of human rights could be dismissed as the subverters of a free society's commitment to the practice of *freedom of religion.* Americans could then look forward breathlessly to the next issues of *Time* and *Newsweek* celebrating the latest breakthrough in *religious research.*

And yet, perhaps it is still not too late to recall that it was respect for the cure of souls, embraced and practiced freely or not at all, that inspired the framers of the Constitution to deprive clerics of secular power. It was enough, I assume they reasoned, that theologians had spiritual power; they needed no other for the discharge of their duties. Similarly, it is respect for the cure of bodies (and "minds"), embraced and practiced freely or not at all, that inspires me to urge that we deprive clinicians of secular power. It is enough, I believe, that physicians have the power inherent in their scientific knowledge and technical skills; they need no other for the discharge of their duties.

Although the essays assembled in this volume have been written over the period of a decade, they are all animated by the aim to explore the ceremonial or religious aspects of various medical practices. Let me hasten to say that I am not denying the scientific or technical aspects of medicine. On the contrary, I believe—and it is rather obvious—that the genuine diagnostic and therapeutic powers of medicine are much greater today than they have ever been in the history of mankind. That, precisely, is why its religious or magical powers are also much greater. Anyone who interprets my efforts to explain, and sometimes to reduce, the magical, religious, and political dimensions of medicine as an effort to cast aspersions on, or to belittle, its scientific and technical dimension does so at his own peril. This book is addressed to those persons who understand the difference between why a priest wears a cassock and a surgeon a sterile gown, between why an orthopedic surgeon uses a cast and a psychoanalyst a couch. Unfortunately, many people don't.

Why don't they? Why indeed should they? Why should anyone want to distinguish between technical and ceremonial acts, roles, and words? There is probably only one reason—namely, the desire to be free and responsible. If a person longs to submit to authority, he will find it useful to bestow ceremonial powers on those who wield technical skills, and vice versa; it will make the authorities seem all the more useful as priests and physicians.

People who possess certain intellectual knowledge or technical skills are obviously superior, at least in those respects, to people who do not. Thus, unless people long for a dictatorship of technicians—say, of physicians—they ought to make sure that the expert's favorable social position due to his having special skills is not further enhanced by attributing ceremonial powers to him as well. Conversely, unless they long to be fooled by fakers—say, by psychiatrists—they ought to make sure that the expert's favorable social position due to his having special ceremonial skills, or to such skills being attributed to him by others, is not further enhanced by crediting him with technical powers he does not possess.

Formerly, people victimized themselves by attributing medical powers to their priests; now, they victimize themselves by attributing magical powers to their physicians. Faced with persons endowed with such superhuman powers—and, of course, benevolence—ordinary men and women are inclined to submit to them with that blind trust whose inexorable consequence is that they make slaves of themselves and tyrants of their "protectors." That is why the framers of the Constitution urged their fellow Americans to respect priests for their faith but to distrust them for their power. To enable them to do so, they erected a wall separating church and state.

I hold, similarly, that people should respect physicians for their skill but should distrust them for their power. But unless the people erect a wall separating medicine and the state, they will be unable to do so and will succumb precisely to that danger from which the First Amendment was supposed to protect them.

# The Theology of Medicine

# 1

# The Moral Physician

What is the moral mandate of medicine? Whom should the physician serve? The answers to these simple questions are by no means clear. Since medicine has rather intimate connections with health and illness, life and death, it is not surprising that we are now as uncertain about the aim of medicine as we are about the aim of life itself. Indeed, we can be no more clear or confident about what medicine is for than we can be about what life is for.

The moral foundations of modern medicine have a dual ancestry: from the Greeks, medicine has inherited the idea that the physician's primary duty is to his patient; and from the Romans, that his primary duty is to do no harm. The first of these ideas, although quite unrealized, is often said to be the ideal of Western medicine; the second, although quite unrealizable, is often said to be its First Commandment.

*Primum non nocere.* (First, do no harm.) What a lofty prescription! But what an absurd one. For the questions immediately arise, To whom should the physician do no harm? and Who will define what constitutes harm?

Life is conflict. The physician often cannot help a person without at the same time harming someone else. He examines an applicant for life insurance, finds that he has diabetes or hypertension, and reports it to the insurance company. He treats a Hitler or Stalin and helps to prolong his life. He declares that a man who tortures his wife with false accusations of infidelity is psychotic and brings about his psychiatric incarceration. In each of these cases, the physician harms someone—either the patient or those in conflict with him. These examples, of course, merely scratch the surface. We may add to them the physician's involvement with persons desiring abortions or narcotics, with suicidal patients, with military organizations, and with research in biological warfare—and we see how woefully inadequate, indeed how utterly useless, are the traditional moral guidelines of medicine for the actual work of the physician, whether as investigator or practitioner. Accordingly, if we wish to confront the moral dilemmas of medicine intelligently, we must start, if not from scratch, then from the basics of ethics and politics.

Everywhere, children, and even many adults, take it for granted not only that there is a god but that he can understand their prayers because he speaks their language. Likewise, children assume that their parents are good, and if their experiences are unbearably inconsistent with that image, they prefer to believe that they themselves are bad rather than that their parents are. The belief that doctors are their patients' agents—serving their patients' interests and needs above all others—seems to me to be of a piece with mankind's basic religious and familial myths. Nor are its roots particularly mysterious: when a person is young, old, or sick, he is handicapped compared with those who are mature and healthy; in the struggle for survival, he will thus inevitably come to depend on his fellows who are relatively unhandicapped.

Such a relationship of dependency is implicit in all situations where clients and experts interact. Because in the case of illness the client fears for his health and for his life, it is especially dramatic and troublesome in medicine. In general, the more dependent a person is on another, the greater will be his need to aggrandize his helper, and the more he aggrandizes his helper, the more dependent he will be on him. The result is that the weak person easily becomes doubly endangered: first, by his weakness and, second, by his dependence on a protector who may choose to harm him. These are the brutal but basic facts of human relationships of which we must never lose sight in considering the ethical problems of biology, medicine, and the healing professions. As helplessness engenders belief in the goodness of the helper, and as utter helplessness engenders belief in his unlimited goodness, those thrust into the roles of helpers—whether as deities or doctors, as priests or politicians—have been only too willing to assent to these characterizations of themselves. This imagery of total virtue and impartial goodness serves not only to mitigate the helplessness of the weak, but also to obscure the conflicts of loyalty to which the protector is subject. Hence, the perennial appeal of the selfless, disinterested helper professing to be the impartial servant of all mankind's needs and interests.

Traditionally, it was, of course, the clergy that claimed to be the agent of all mankind—asserting that they were the servants of God, the creator and caretaker of all mankind. Although this absurd claim had its share of success, it was doomed to be rejected in time because the representatives of the most varied creeds all claimed to speak for the whole of mankind. Gullible as men are, they can stand just so much inconsistency. Thus, by the time our so-called modern age rolled around, the mythology of any particular religion speaking for all of mankind became exposed for what it is—the representation of certain values and interests as the values and interests of everyone. Nietzsche called this the death of God. But God did not die; He merely disappeared behind the stage of history to don other robes and reemerged as scientist and doctor.

Since the seventeenth century, it has been mainly the scientist, and especially the so-called medical scientist or physician, who has claimed to owe his allegiance, not to his profession or nation or religion, but to all of mankind. But if I am right in insisting that such a claim is always and of necessity a sham—that mankind is so large and heterogeneous a group, consisting of members with inherently conflicting values and interests, that it is meaningless to claim allegiance to it or to its interests—then it behooves us as independent thinkers to ask ourselves, "Whose agent is the expert?"

Plato is fond of using the physician as his model of the rational ruler, and in *The Republic* he explicitly considers the question of whose agent the physician is. Early in that dialogue he offers us this exchange between Socrates and Thrasymachus:

> Now tell me about the physician in that strict sense you spoke of: is it his business to earn money or to treat his patients? Remember, I mean your physician who is worthy of the name?
> To treat his patients.[1]

It would seem that we have not advanced one step beyond this naïve, hortatory answer to the question of whose agent the physician is. In the conventional contemporary view too, the doctor's role is seen as consisting in the prevention and treatment of his patient's illness. But such an answer leaves out of account the crucial question of who defines health and illness, prevention and treatment.

Although Plato seemingly supports the idea that the physician's duty is to be his patient's agent, as we shall see that is not what he supports at all. By making the physician the definer not only of his own but also of his patient's best interests, Plato actually supports a coercive-collectivistic medical ethic rather than an autonomous-individualistic one.

Here is how Plato develops his defense of the physician as agent of the state:

> But now take the art of medicine itself. . . . [It] does not study its own interests, but the needs of the body, just as a groom shows his skill by caring for horses, not for the art of grooming. And so every art seeks, not its own advantage—for it has no deficiencies—but the interest of the subject on which it is exercised.[2]

Having established his claim for benevolent altruism, Plato proceeds to draw the ethical and political conclusions he was aiming at all along: the moral justification of the control of the subordinate by the superior—patient by doctor, subject by ruler:

> But surely, Thrasymachus, every art has authority and superior power over its subject. . . . So far as the arts are concerned, then, no art ever studies or enjoins the interest of the superior party, but always that of the weaker over which it has authority. . . . So the physician, as such, studies only the patient's interest, not his own. For as we agreed, the business of the physician, in the strict sense, is not to make money for himself, but to exercise his power over the patient's body. . . . And so

1. *The Republic of Plato,* trans. F. M. Cornford (New York: Oxford University Press, 1945), p. 22.
2. Ibid., p. 23.

> with government of any kind: no ruler, in so far as he is acting as ruler, will study or enjoin what is for his own interest. All that he says and does will be said and done with a view to what is good and proper for the subject for whom he practices his art.[3]

That this argument is contrary to the facts Thrasymachus himself points out. But such facts scarcely affect the force of Plato's rhetoric, which is based on the perpetually recurring passions of men and women to control and be controlled. Thus, Plato's rhetoric still has an astonishingly timely ring: it could serve, without any significant modification, as a contemporary exposition of what is now usually called medical ethics.

Indeed, so little have men's views changed in the past twenty-five hundred years on the dilemma of the physician's dual allegiance, to himself and to his patient, that it will be worth our while to follow to its end Plato's argument about the selflessness of the moral man of medicine:

> . . . any kind of authority, in the state or in private life, must, in its character of authority, consider solely what is best for those under its care. . . . each [skill] brings us some benefit that is peculiar to it: medicine gives health, for example; the art of navigation, safety at sea; and so on.
>
> Yes.
>
> And wage-earning brings us wages; that is its distinctive product. Now, speaking with that precision which you proposed, you would not say that the art of navigation is the same as the art of medicine, merely on the ground that a ship's captain regained his health on a voyage, because the sea air was good for him. No more would you identify the practice of medicine with wage-earning because a man may keep his health while earning wages, or a physician attending a case may receive a fee.
>
> No.
>
> . . . This benefit, then—the receipt of wages—does not come to a man from his special art. If we are to speak strictly, the physician, as such, produces health; the builder, a house; and then each, in his further capacity as wage-earner, gets his pay. . . . Well, then, Thrasymachus, it is now clear that no form of skill or authority provides for its own benefit.[4]

3. Ibid., pp. 23–24.
4. Ibid., pp. 27–28.

As these quotations show, Plato is a paternalist.[5] Quite simply, what Plato advocates is what many people seem to need or want, at least some of the time: namely, that the expert should be a leader who takes the burden of responsibility for personal choice off the shoulders of the ordinary man or woman who is his client. This ethical ideal and demand, characteristic of the closed society, must be contrasted with the ethical ideal and demand of the open society, in which the expert must speak the truth and the client must bear the responsibility of his own existence—including his choice of expert.

I shall have more to say later about the fundamental alternative between authority and autonomy, noble lies and painful truths. For now, I want to follow Plato a little further in *The Republic* to show how inextricably intertwined in his thought are the notions of authority and mendacity—indeed, how it is power that renders lying virtuous and powerlessness that renders it wicked:

> Is the spoken falsehood always a hateful thing? Is it not sometimes helpful—in war, for instance, or as a sort of medicine? . . . And in those legends we were discussing just now, we can turn fiction to account; not knowing the facts about the distant past, we can make our fiction as good an embodiment of truth as possible.[6]

In the Platonic program of fictionalizing history, we recognize, of course, another much-applauded modern scientific enterprise—in fact, a species of psychiatric prevarication that its practitioners pretentiously call *psychohistory*. As the modern psychiatric physician is entitled, by his limitless benevolence, to use mendacity as medicine, so, according to Plato, is the ruler:

> If we were right in saying that gods have no use for falsehood and it is useful to mankind only in the way of a medicine, obviously a medicine should be handled by no one but a physician. . . . If anyone, then, is to practice deception, either on the country's enemies or on its citizens, it must be the Rulers of the commonwealth, acting for its benefit; no one else may meddle with this privilege. For a private

5. See K. R. Popper, *The Open Society and Its Enemies* (Princeton, N.J.: Princeton University Press, 1950).
6. *The Republic*, p. 74.

> person to mislead such Rulers we shall declare to be a worse offense than for a patient to mislead his doctor. . . .[7]

Plato also uses the metaphor of mendacity as a medicine to justify his eugenic policies. All the mischief done ever since in the name of genetics as a means of improving the human race has been perpetrated by following the policy here proposed by Plato:

> Anything like unregulated unions would be a profanation in a state whose citizens lead the good life. The Rulers will not allow such a thing. . . . We shall need consummate skill in our Rulers . . . because they will have to administer a large dose of that medicine we spoke of earlier. . . . We said, if you remember, that such expedients would be useful as a sort of medicine. . . . It follows from what we have just said that, if we are to keep our flock at the highest pitch of excellence, there should be as many unions of the best of both sexes, and as few of the inferior, as possible, and that only the offspring of the better unions should be kept. And again, no one but the Rulers must know how all this is being effected; otherwise, our herd of Guardians may become rebellious.[8]

Clearly, the Platonic physician is an agent of the state—and, if need be, the adversary of his patient. In view of the immense influence of Platonic ideas on modern medicine, it is hardly surprising that we now face moral dilemmas attributable directly to the medical arrangement advocated by Plato and his countless loyal supporters, past and present.

Lest it seem that I have overemphasized the Platonic physician's allegiance to the state, even at the cost of his being the unconcealed adversary of the so-called patient, let us see what Plato says about physicians qua physicians, not as the models for rulers. What he says may seem shocking to some of us—because it sounds so modern and because it supports the most disreputable medical, eugenic, and psychiatric policies of twentieth-century governments, both totalitarian and free.

Revealingly Plato begins his discussion of the duties of doctors by reviling malingerers and persons now usually called mentally ill. Plato's objection to medicalizing ordinary miseries—problems in

7. Ibid., p. 78.
8. Ibid., pp. 157–159.

living—is, to be sure, a position I myself support, but for a reason and an aim that are the very opposite of his: he wants doctors to persecute such people, and persecuted by them they have been; whereas I want doctors to leave them alone if that is what the patients want.[9]

> Is it not [asks Plato rhetorically] also disgraceful to need doctoring, not merely for a wound or an attack of some seasonal disorder, but because, through living in idleness and luxury, our bodies are infested with winds and humours, like marsh gas in a stagnant pool, so that the sons of Asclepius are put to inventing for diseases such ingenious names as flatulence and catarrh?
>
> Yes; they are queer, these modern terms.
>
> And not in use, I fancy, in the days of Asclepius himself. . . . in the old days, until the time of Herodicus, the sons of Asclepius had no use for the modern coddling treatment of disease. But Herodicus, who was a gymnastic teacher who lost his health, combined training and doctoring in such a way as to become a plague to himself first and foremost and to many others after him.
>
> How?
>
> By lingering out his death. He had a mortal disease, and he spent all his life at its beck and call, with no hope of a cure and no time for anything but doctoring himself. . . . his skill only enabled him to reach old age in a prolonged death struggle.[10]

Plato clearly disapproves of such use of medicine and the art of the physician. And he minces no words in asserting that a physician ministering to a sufferer such as Herodicus is a bad man—a traitor to the community and the state.

> If Asclepius did not reveal these valetudinarian arts to his descendants, it was not from ignorance or lack of experience, but because he realized that in every well-ordered community each man has his ap-

9. See especially my *The Myth of Mental Illness: Foundations of a Theory of Personal Conduct*, rev. ed. (New York: Harper & Row, 1974), *The Manufacture of Madness: A Comparative Study of the Inquisition and the Mental Health Movement* (New York: Harper & Row, 1970), and *The Ethics of Psychoanalysis: The Theory and Method of Autonomous Psychotherapy* (New York: Basic Books, 1964).

10. *The Republic*, pp. 95–96.

> pointed task which he must perform; no one has leisure to spend all his life in being ill and doctoring himself.[11]

What then should a chronically ill person do? He should die—"get rid of his troubles by dying"[12] is the way Plato puts it—for his own sake and the sake of the state. But what about people who feel sick, who are preoccupied by their own ill health and its care, but who are not sick enough to die? Physicians should turn their backs on such people. "They should not be treated,"[13] he says, thus unmistakably identifying the sufferer's own desire for medical care as a wholly irrelevant criterion for legitimizing such treatment.

It seems to me that never before—not just in totalitarian societies but in all societies—has Western medicine been so dangerously close to realizing this particular Platonic ideal as today. Here again are Plato's words on the subject:

> Surely, there could be no worse hindrance than this excessive care of the body. . . . Shall we say, then, that Asclepius recognized this and revealed the art of medicine for the benefit of people of sound constitution who normally led a healthy life, but had contracted some definite ailment? He would rid them of their disorders by means of drugs or the knife and tell them to go on living as usual, so as not to impair their usefulness as citizens. But where the body was diseased through and through, he would not try, by nicely calculated evacuations and doses, to prolong a miserable existence and let his patient beget children who were likely to be as sickly as himself. Treatment, he thought, would be wasted on a man who could not live in his ordinary round of duties and was consequently useless to himself and society.[14]

Implicit throughout this dialogue is the identity of the person making the judgment about who is useful and who is not, who should be treated and who should not be: it is the physician, not the patient.

Herein lie the main lessons for our present ethical predicaments in genetics; they are best framed as questions: Do we support or op-

11. Ibid., p. 96.
12. Ibid.
13. Ibid., p. 98.
14. Ibid., p. 97.

pose the view—and the policy—that the expert's role should be limited to providing truthful information to his client? Do we support or oppose the view—and the policy—that the expert's duty is to decide how the nonexperts should live and that he should therefore be provided with the power to impose his policies on those so unenlightened as to reject them?

If we are not skilled at analyzing Plato's arguments, if we do not realize that choices such as these confront us with the necessity of ranking our priorities, and if we blind ourselves to the conflicts in life between bodily health and personal freedom, then we may become geniuses at manipulating the gene but will remain morons about trying to manipulate our fellow man and letting him manipulate us. Plato had, of course, no hesitation in judging, and in letting physicians judge, whose life was worth something and whose was not, who should be treated and who should not:

> . . . if a man had a sickly constitution and intemperate habits, his life was worth nothing to himself or to anyone else; medicine was not meant for such people and they should not be treated, though they might be richer than Midas.[15]

It seems to me difficult to overemphasize that Plato's foregoing proposals are political remedies for perennial moral problems. How should society treat the sick and the weak, the old and the "socially useless"? How should the services of healers be employed—like those of soldiers, of priests, or of entrepreneurs? We should beware of flattering ourselves by believing that new biomedical capabilities necessarily generate genuinely new moral problems, especially since we haven't solved—haven't even faced—our old problems.

I shall not belabor here the idiocies and horrors proposed or perpetrated in the name of medicine, and specifically genetics, in recent decades. A single example should suffice to illustrate my point—that medical experts, like all human beings, may easily identify themselves with the holders of power, may eagerly become their obedient servants, and may in this way suggest and support the most heinous policies of mayhem and murder against suffering or stigmatized individuals.

15. Ibid., p. 98.

The following words, written in 1939, are not those of a Nazi physician, but of a distinguished scientist who must have been thoroughly familiar with Plato:

> Eugenics is indispensable for the perpetuation of the strong. A great race must propagate its best elements. . . . Women [however] voluntarily deteriorate through alcohol and tobacco. They subject themselves to dangerous dietary regimens in order to obtain a conventional slenderness of their figure. Besides, they refuse to bear children. Such a defection is due to their education, to the progress of feminism, to the growth of short-sighted selfishness. . . .
>
> Eugenics may exercise a great influence upon the destiny of the civilized races. . . . The propagation of the insane and the feebleminded . . . must be prevented. . . . No criminal causes so much misery in a human group as the tendency to insanity. . . . Obviously, those who are afflicted with a heavy ancestral burden of insanity, feeble-mindedness, or cancer should not marry. . . . Thus, eugenics asks for the sacrifice of many individuals. . . .
>
> . . . Women should receive a higher education, not in order to become doctors, lawyers, or professors, but to rear their offspring to be valuable human beings.
>
> There remains the unsolved problem of the immense number of defectives and criminals. . . . As already pointed out, gigantic sums are now required to maintain prisons and insane asylums and protect the public against gangsters and lunatics. Why do we preserve these useless and harmful beings? The abnormal prevent the development of the normal. . . . Why should society not dispose of the criminals and the insane in a more economical manner? . . . Criminality and insanity can be prevented only by a better knowledge of man, by eugenics, by changes in education and in social conditions. Meanwhile, criminals have to be dealt with effectively. . . . The conditioning of petty criminals with the whip, or some more scientific procedure, followed by a short stay in hospital, would probably suffice to insure order. Those who have murdered, robbed while armed with automatic pistol or machine gun, kidnapped children, despoiled the poor of their savings, misled the public in important matters, should be humanely and economically disposed of in small euthanasic institutions supplied with proper gases. A similar treatment could be advantageously applied to the insane, guilty of criminal acts.[16]

16. A. Carrel, *Man, the Unknown* (New York: Harper & Row, 1939), pp. 299–302, 318–319.

The man who wrote this was Alexis Carrel (1873–1944), surgeon and biologist, member of the Rockefeller Institute in New York, and the recipient in 1912 of the Nobel Prize in physiology and medicine for his work on suturing blood vessels.

Besides being his own agent, which of course the medical scientist or physician always is, and besides being an agent of his patient, which the physician is more and more rarely (hence the disenchantment with medical care among both physicians and patients despite the remarkable technical advances of medical science), the physician may be—and indeed often is—the agent of every conceivable social institution or group. It could hardly be otherwise. Social institutions are composed of, and cater to, the needs of human beings; and among human needs, the need for the health of those inside the group—and frequently for the sickness of those outside of it—is paramount. Hence, the physician is enlisted, and has always been enlisted, to help some persons and harm others—his injurious activities being defined, as we have already seen in Plato's *Republic*, as helping the state or some other institution.

Let me offer a very brief review of how physicians have through the ages not only helped some, usually those who supported the dominant social ethic, but also harmed others, usually those who opposed the dominant social ethic.

During the late Middle Ages, physicians were prominent in the Inquisition, helping the inquisitors to ferret out witches by appropriate "diagnostic" examinations and tests.[17]

The so-called discipline of public health, originating in what was first revealingly called "medical police" (*Medizinalpolizei*), came into being to serve the interests of the absolutist rulers of seventeenth- and eighteenth-century Europe. The term, according to George Rosen, was first employed in 1764 by Wolfgang Thomas Rau (1721–1772):

> This idea of medical police, that is, the creation of a medical policy by government and its implementation through administrative regulation, rapidly achieved popularity. Efforts were made to apply this

17. See *The Myth of Mental Illness*, pp. 32–34.

concept to the major health problems of the period, which reached a high point in the work of Johann Peter Frank (1748–1821) and Franz Anton Mai (1742–1814).[18]

The medical police were never intended to help the individual citizen or sick patient; instead, they were quite explicitly designed "to secure for the monarch and the state increased power and wealth."[19] Since increased power and wealth for the state could often be obtained only at the expense of decreased health and freedom for certain citizens, we witness here a collision between the Platonic and Hippocratic medical ethics—the former easily triumphing over the latter. Rosen's summary of Frank's work shows its undisguisedly Platonic character:

> Carrying out the idea that the health of the people is the responsibility of the state, Frank presented a system of public and private hygiene, worked out in minute detail. . . . A spirit of enlightenment and humanitarianism is clearly perceptible throughout the entire work, but as might be expected from a public medical official who spent his life in the service of various absolute rulers, great and small, the exposition serves not so much for the instruction of the people, or even of physicians, as for the guidance of officials who are supposed to regulate and supervise for the benefit of society all the spheres of human activity, even those most personal. Frank is a representative of enlightened despotism. The modern reader may, in many instances, be repelled by his excessive reliance on legal regulation, and by the minuteness of detail with which Frank worked out his proposals, especially in questions of individual, personal hygiene.[20]

Among Frank's more interesting proposals was a tax on bachelors—part of the medical police's effort to increase the population to provide more soldiers for the monarch—a proposal we have still not ceased implementing.

The French Revolution helped to cement further the alliance between medicine and the state. This alliance is symbolized by the healer's aspiring to perfect more humane methods of execution. In

18. G. Rosen, *A History of Public Health* (New York: MD Publications, 1958), pp. 161–162.
19. G. Rosen, "Cameralism and the Concept of Medical Police," *Bulletin of the History of Medicine* 27 (1953): 42.
20. Rosen, *A History of Public Health*, p. 162.

1792, the guillotine—developed and named after Dr. Joseph Ignace Guillotin, a physician and member of the Revolutionary Assembly and creator of its Health Committee (*Comité de salubrité*)—became the official instrument of execution in France. Again, it is revealing that the first guillotine was assembled at the Bicêtre, one of Paris's famous insane asylums, and that it was tried out on live sheep and then on three cadavers of patients from the asylum. After the first flush of enthusiasm for this medical advance wore off, Guillotin's contribution to human welfare was viewed, even in those days, ambivalently—leading him to remark in his last will, "It is difficult to do good to men without causing oneself some unpleasantness."[21]

In our own day, in the so-called free societies, virtually every group or agency, public and private, has enlisted the physician as an agent of its particular interests. The school and the factory, employers and labor unions, airlines and insurance companies, immigration authorities and drug-control agencies, prisons and mental hospitals, all employ physicians. The physician so employed has a choice only between being a loyal agent of his employer, serving his employer's interests as the latter defines them, or being a disloyal agent of his employer, serving interests other than his employer's as the physician himself defines them.

The principal moral decision for the physician who does not work in an ideal private-practice situation is choosing what organization or institution he shall work for; more than anything else, that will determine the sort of moral agent he can be to his patient and others. It follows from this that we should pay more attention than has been our habit to the ways institutions and organizations—whether the CIA or the United Nations or any other prestigious and powerful group—use medical knowledge and skills. Although these considerations may seem simple, their appreciation is not reflected by what seems to be the viewpoint that characterizes the recent burgeoning of literature on problems of medical ethics, especially as they relate to genetics. To illustrate this, let me quote two remarks from an international conference in 1971 on Ethical Issues in Human

21. Quoted in A. Soubiran, *The Good Doctor Guillotin and His Strange Device*, trans. M. McGraw (London: Souvenir Press, 1963), p. 214.

Genetics, devoted mainly to problems of genetic knowledge and counseling.

One participant, a professor of genetics in Paris, in a discussion about counseling parents who might give birth to a child with Tay-Sachs disease, had this to say:

> I think the question is whether I would like to suppress a child or not. My simple answer is definitely not, because we have to recognize one thing which is very frequently overlooked: medicine is essentially and by nature working against natural selection. That is the reason why medicine was invented. It was really to fight in the contrary sense of natural selection. . . . When medicine is used to reinforce natural selection, it is no longer medicine; it is eugenics. It doesn't matter if the work is palatable or not; that is what it is.[22]

There are two things seriously wrong here. First, this expert's remarks about the antagonism between medicine and natural selection are nonsense—and remarkable nonsense at that for a biologist to entertain and expound. Second, by speaking about "suppressing a child," this expert equates and confuses advising a parent not to have a child, performing an abortion, and killing an infant.

Another participant, a professor of sociology in Ithaca, New York, in a discussion of the "Implications of Parental Diagnosis for the Quality of, and Right to, Human Life," said:

> . . . the best way of expressing its [society's] interest is through the counselor-physician, who in effect has a dual responsibility to the individual whom he serves and to the society of which he and she are parts. . . . we will all certainly be diminished as human beings, if not in great moral peril, if we allow ourselves to accept abortion for what are essentially trivial reasons. On the other hand, we will, I fear, be in equal danger if we don't accept abortion as one means of ensuring that both the quantity and quality of the human race are kept within reasonable limits.[23]

22. J. Lejeune, "Discussion" of F. C. Fraser's "Survey of Counseling Practices," in B. Hilton et al., eds., *Ethical Issues in Human Genetics: Genetic Counseling and the Use of Genetic Knowledge* (New York: Plenum, 1973), p. 19.

23. R. S. Morison, "Implications of Prenatal Diagnosis for the Quality of, and Right to, Human Life: Society as a Standard," in ibid., pp. 210–211.

If that is how the experts reason about the ethical problems of genetics, we are in a bad way indeed. The priest, the accountant, and the defense lawyer do not try to serve antagonistic interests simultaneously; the politician, the psychiatrist, and the expert on genetic counseling do.[24]

My views on medical ethics in general and on the ethical implications of genetic knowledge and engineering in particular may be summarized as follows.

The biologist and the physician are, first and foremost, individuals; as individuals they have their own moral values that they are likely to try to realize in their professional work as well as their private lives.

In general, we should regard the medical man, whether as investigator or practitioner, as the agent of the party that pays him and thus controls him; whether he helps or harms the so-called patient thus depends not so much on whether he is a good or bad man as on whether the function of the institution whose agent he is, is to help or harm the so-called patient.

Insofar as the biologist or physician chooses to act as a scientist, he has an unqualified obligation to tell the truth; he cannot compromise that obligation without disqualifying himself as a scientist. In actual practice, only certain kinds of situations permit the medical man to fulfill such an unqualified obligation to truth telling.

Insofar as the biologist or physician chooses to act as a social engineer, he is an agent of the particular moral and political values he espouses and tries to realize or of those his employer espouses and tries to realize.

The biologist's or physician's claim that he represents disinterested abstract values—such as mankind, health, or treatment—should be disallowed; and his efforts to balance, and his claim to represent, multiple conflicting interests—such as those of the fetus against the mother or society or of the individual against the family or the state—should be exposed for what they conceal, perhaps his secret loyalty to one of the conflicting parties or his cynical re-

24. See my *Ideology and Insanity: Essays on the Psychiatric Dehumanization of Man* (Garden City, N.Y.: Doubleday, Anchor Press, 1973), esp. pp. 190–217.

jection of the interests of both parties in favor of his own self-aggrandizement.

If we value personal freedom and dignity, we should, in confronting the moral dilemmas of biology, genetics, and medicine, insist that the expert's allegiance to the agents and values he serves be made explicit and that the power inherent in his specialized knowledge and skill not be accepted as justification for his exercising specific controls over those lacking such knowledge and skill.

# 2

# Illness and Indignity

All of us in the health professions share certain fundamental aspirations and goals, among which the most important are keeping the healthy person healthy, restoring the sick person to health, and most generally, safeguarding and prolonging life. That these ends are so overwhelmingly good and noble is what makes their pursuit so gratifying and those in the health professions so richly honored and rewarded.

But life would be simpler than it is if health and longevity were its only, or even its principal, purposes—that is, if there were no goals or values that often conflict with their pursuit. One of the values that we cherish, and that often conflicts with the pursuit of health at any cost, is dignity.

Dignity is of course that ineffable and yet obvious quality of human encounters that enriches the participants' self-esteem. The process of dignification is characteristically reciprocal; dignified conduct in one person or party generates dignified conduct in another and vice versa.

Conversely, indignity is that equally obvious but much more easily definable quality of human encounters that impoverishes the participants' self-esteem. There are many forms of it, one of the most common and most tragic being the indignity of disability, illness, and old age. Many sick people behave, simply because of their illness, in ways that make their conduct undignified. When a person loses control over his basic bodily functions, when he cannot work, then—often against his most intense efforts—he is rendered undignified. Language, the oldest but still the most reliable guide to a people's true sentiments, starkly reveals the intimate connection between illness and indignity. In English, we use the same word to describe an expired passport, an indefensible argument, an illegitimate legal document, and a person disabled by disease. We call each of them *invalid*. To be an invalid, then, is to be an invalidated person, a human being stamped *not valid* by the invisible but invincible hand of popular opinion. While invalidism carries with it the heaviest burden of indignity, some of the stigma adheres to virtually all illness, to virtually any participation in the role of patient.

This fact generates two very important problems for people in the health professions: one is that the sick person's undignified behavior may stimulate the professional person's inclination to respond with undignified behavior of his own; the other is that patients disabled in ways that render them grossly undignified may prefer death with dignity to life without it. Let me offer a few observations on each of these problems.

The connections between illness and indignity are, in the main, quite obvious. Because the patient cannot work, cannot take care of himself, must disrobe and submit his body for examination by strangers, and for many other equally good reasons, the sick person perceives himself as suffering not only from an illness but also from a loss of dignity. Moreover, the patient's loss of dignity often generates a reciprocal loss of respect for him by those around him, especially by his family and physicians. This unfortunate process of degradation is often concealed, though in my opinion never very successfully, by the imagery and vocabulary of paternalism—family and physician treating the patient as if he were a child (or childlike) and the patient treating them as if they were his parents (or superiors).

This fundamental tendency—to infantilize the sick person and to parentalize the healer—manifests itself in countless ways in the everyday practice of medicine. For example, the patient is expected to trust his physician, but the physician need not trust his patient; the patient is expected to impart his intimate bodily and personal experiences to the physician, but the physician may withhold vital information from the patient.

The patient's undignified position vis-à-vis the medical authorities is symbolized by the linguistic structure of the medical situation. The patient communicates in ordinary language, which he shares with his physician; the physician communicates partly in the same language, insofar as he speaks *to* his patient, and partly in another language, insofar as he speaks *about* him. The physician's second language used to be Latin and is now the technical jargon of medicine. The upshot is that patients often do not know or understand what is wrong with them, what is in their medical records, or what drugs they are taking. To be sure, like children or other fearful, humiliated, or oppressed persons, patients often do not want to know these things. Yet even if this were so—and it is not always so—it would not, in my opinion, justify withholding such information from them. After all, many people do not want to know what is under the hood of an automobile, but we would not accept that as justifying automobile manufacturers in maintaining a systematic policy of withholding this information from car buyers or releasing it to them only under special circumstances.

My point is that many people today accept it as right and proper that patients should not understand their prescriptions or that they should not know what is in their hospital records; at the same time, they object to the indignities that the medical situation often imposes on them. The result of this unarticulated conflict is that people often feel anxious and humiliated at the prospect of seeking medical care and frequently avoid or reject such care altogether.

We must keep in mind that people want and need not only health but also dignity, that often they can obtain health only at the cost of dignity, and that sometimes they prefer not to pay that price. It is obvious, for example, that patients participate most eagerly and most intelligently in medical situations that entail little or no humiliation on their part; thus, people seek help freely for refractive errors of their eyes or for athletic injuries. It is equally obvious that patients participate most reluctantly or not at all in those medical situations that entail a great deal of humiliation on their part; thus, people are often reluctant to seek medical help for syphilis or gonorrhea, even though these diseases can now be treated effectively and safely, and they often do not seek medical help at all for "conditions" whose treatment is humiliating to the point of legally articulated stigmatization—such as drug addiction or the so-called psychoses.

There is a practical lesson here for all of us—namely, that it is not enough that we do a technically competent job of healing the patient's body; we must do an equally competent job of safeguarding his dignity and self-esteem. In proportion as we fail in this latter task, we destroy the practical value of our technical competence for the sick person.

Inexorably, efforts to combat disease or stave off death conflict with the need to maintain dignity. The currently popular phrase *death with dignity* is therefore quite misleading: it is not just that people want to die with dignity, but rather that they want to live with it. After all, dying is a part of life, not of death. It is precisely because many people live without dignity that they also die without it. Determined and dignified persons, whether soldiers or surgeons, have always wanted to die with their boots on. Military men have traditionally preferred death on the battlefield or even suicide to surrender and loss of face; medical men prefer a sudden death from a myocardial infarct to a lingering demise from generalized carcinomatosis. These examples illustrate my contention that there is often an irreconcilable antagonism between preserving and promoting dignity and preserving and promoting health.

There are of course many such antagonisms in life, which is what makes human existence tragic in the classical Greek and Christian conceptions of it. For example, in personal and political affairs, we desire both freedom and security but can often gain the one only at the expense of the other. The modern scientific and technical outlook, valuable through it is for realizing scientific and technical ends, misleads us badly insofar as it deals in isolation with the concepts of health and dignity and promises to maximize each at the cost of nothing more than scientific and technical effort and expertise. This perspective has led to a lopsided—and, indeed, erroneous—estimate of the bargain entailed in maintaining or securing good health. Many people now believe—and they are grievously mistaken—that they can retain or recover their health merely as a result of scientific advances in medicine (fashionably called *breakthroughs*) without their having to make any sacrifices for it—that is, without their having to pay money for it, without their having to curb their appetites and passions for it, and without their having to suffer some loss of dignity for it.

The irreconcilable conflict that may arise between prolonging life and maintaining dignity was—as were all the fundamental conflicts characteristic of the human condition—well appreciated and articulated by the ancient Greeks. In the *Phaedo*, Plato illustrates this dilemma and Socrates' method of resolving it.

The death scene opens with Socrates and some of his closest friends gathered in anticipation of Socrates' drinking the hemlock. After some conversation between Socrates and his friends, Socrates says farewell and asks the executioner to bring the poisoned cup. But Crito urges Socrates to wait, to prolong his life for as long as he can: "But Socrates," he pleads, ". . . I know that other men take the poison quite late, and eat and drink heartily, and even enjoy the company of their chosen friends, after the announcement has been made. So do not hurry; there is still time."[1]

Socrates' reply articulates the distinction between life as a biological process that may and perhaps ought to be prolonged for as long as possible and as a spiritual pilgrimage that can and should be traversed and ended in a proper manner. This is what Socrates says:

> And those whom you speak of, Crito, naturally do so; for they think that they will be gainers by so doing. And I naturally shall not do so; for I think that I should gain nothing by drinking the poison a little later but my own contempt for so greedily saving up a life which is already spent.[2]

The distinction between the death of the body and the end of life, which is the difference between Crito's and Socrates' outlook on life and death, continues to baffle us in the health sciences. The main reason why it does is, remarkably, also explained by Socrates.

Crito asks his friend how he wants to be buried. Socrates replies:

1. Plato, *Euthyphro, Apology, Crito, with the Death Scene from Phaedo*, trans. F. J. Church, (Indianapolis, Ind.: Bobbs-Merrill, 1956), p. 69.
2. Ibid.

> He [Crito] thinks that I am the body which he will presently see as a corpse, and he asks me how he is to bury me. All the arguments which I have used to prove that I shall not remain with you after I have drunk the poison . . . have been thrown away on him. . . . For, dear Crito, you must know that to use words wrongly is not only a fault in itself, it also corrupts the soul. You must be of good cheer, and say that you are burying my body; and you may bury it as you please, and you think right.[3]

The distinction Socrates here makes between himself and his body is at once obvious and elusive; we all know how often modern people, scientifically informed and enlightened people, fail to make this distinction.

The richness of the death scene for our theme is by no means exhausted by my foregoing remarks on it. There is significance, too, in Socrates' parting words. "Crito," he says, "I owe a cock to Asclepius; do not forget it."[4] The ritual sacrifice Socrates here requests his friend to make on his behalf refers to the custom of offering, on recovering from sickness, a cock to Asclepius, the god of healing. In other words, Socrates views his death as a recovery from an illness, presaging the Christian view.

In short, the message I want to bring to you is simply this: Do your utmost to exercise your skills in healing, but do not do so by sacrificing dignity, either your patient's or your own—the two being tied together by bonds not unlike those of matrimony, except, especially in these days, stronger. For, if I may paraphrase the Scriptures, what does it profit a man if he gains his health but loses his dignity?

3. Ibid., p. 68.
4. Ibid., p. 70.

# 3

# A Map for Medical Ethics: The Moral Justifications of Medical Interventions

After a lifetime of reflection on what it means to be a patient and to be sick, and what it means to be a doctor and to treat, it has finally dawned on me that much of our contemporary confusion concerning medical ethics rests on our failure to articulate the differences between certain fundamental facts and certain elementary justifications and to agree on which considerations justify certain medical interventions and which do not. In this brief essay, I shall try to offer a map that may help us to orient ourselves in the maze of medico-ethical problems that now face us. Like any map, it will not tell us where we ought to go. But it will tell us where the various roads lead.

Let us choose as our paradigm of illness breast cancer and as our paradigm of treatment removal of the cancerous breast. Cancer is an illness; that is a biological and medical fact. Mastectomy is a treatment; that is a surgical and legal fact. The medico-ethical and medico-legal question is, What justifies the medical (surgical) intervention of mastectomy?

1. According to some people, such a patient should have a mastectomy because she has cancer. That is the disease-oriented justification for the intervention.

2. According to others, she should have a mastectomy because it will cure her. That is the treatment-oriented justification for the intervention.

3. And according to still others, she may have a mastectomy because she seeks medical help, the physician offers surgical treatment, and the surgeon has recommended and the patient has agreed to a mastectomy. That is the consent-oriented justification for the intervention.

It is important to keep in mind that although in the ideal case the three justifications coincide and collapse, as it were, into a single affirmation by both patient and doctor about what ought to be done, the justifications are independent of one another and often in conflict. A few illustrations will exemplify and dramatize the potential disjunctions between the medical facts and the moral justifications considered thus far.

1. Disease may not justify medical intervention—for example, if the patient rejects treatment because she or he is a Christian Scientist (or for any other reason). And medical intervention may be justified in the absence of disease: abortion and vasectomy are medical interventions, but pregnancy and the capacity to impregnate are not diseases.

2. Cure (in the sense of therapeutic effectiveness) may not justify medical intervention—for example, as before, if the patient rejects the treatment. And medical intervention may be justified in the absence of therapeutic effectiveness: venesection was, and electroshock is, an accepted form of treatment—however, we now acknowledge that bloodletting only impaired the patient's circulatory system, and we may one day acknowledge that electrically induced convulsions only impair the patient's central nervous system.

3. Consent may not legally justify medical intervention—for example, if the patient is a morphine addict and the physician supplies him with morphine. And medical intervention may legally be justified in the absence of consent—for example, if electroshock is given to a so-called suicidally depressed commited mental patient.

Thus, our dilemmas of medical ethics have at least two sources: factual (or epistemological) and moral (or ethical). In the former class belong such questions as, What is disease? What is treatment? What is consent? In the latter belongs the question, What justifies certain particular contacts between sufferers and healers that we call medical (surgical, psychiatric, and so on) interventions?

There are vexing problems in both categories. How do we define, know, or agree on what is disease or treatment? Is pregnancy (wanted or unwanted) a disease? Is abortion a treatment? Is old age a disease? Is euthanasia a treatment? The problems are obvious, and there is no need to belabor them here. Suffice it to say that even if we agreed—which would not make us right—on what we shall count as falling into these classes and outside of them, many of our medico-ethical problems would remain unaffectedly vexing. For regardless of our agreement on matters of definition, naming, or "factualness," there would remain our problems concerning justification. Those problems require choosing and accepting responsibility for the inexorable consequences of our choices.

We have several choices with respect to justifying medical interventions. First, we might travel west (as it were)—that is, justify medical intervention by disease. That way lie the coercions and countercoercions of patients and doctors, physicians and politicians. For if disease justifies treatment, then individuals will tend to claim or conceal diseases depending on whether or not they want particular treatments. And medical professionals will tend to discover or deny diseases depending on whether they want to impose or withhold particular treatments. (People who claim to be in severe pain in order to obtain analgesics and physicians who impose methadone on those who desire heroin are signposts down that road.)

Second, we might travel east—that is, justify medical intervention by treatment. That way lie the similar coercions and countercoercions of patients and doctors, physicians and politicians. For if curative efficacy justifies medical intervention, physicians will tend to claim or conceal therapeutic powers depending on whether or not they want to dispense it, impose it, or withhold it. And individuals will tend, depending on their desires, to try to qualify for, or disqualify themselves from, various treatments. (Physicians who avoid the use and falsify the pharmacological properties of opiates, psychiatrists who claim to be able to treat mental illness by imprisonment, and politicians who legislate about the imprisoned mental patient's rights to treatment are signposts down that road.)

Third, we might travel north—that is, justify medical intervention by consent. That way—where the air is clear but cool—lies medicine as a contractual service occupation. In such a system, only those patients who want treatment will receive it and only those physicians who want to dispense treatment will administer it. This system will make possible certain medical interventions that please patient and doctor but may displease others; and it will make impossible certain others desired by the patient, the patient's family, the doctor, the medical profession, or society generally, because one or another or both of the parties necessary for the medical contract refuse to enter into it. (Individuals with infectious diseases such as gonorrhea who refuse treatment or Catholic physicians who refuse to do abortions are signposts down that road.)

Finally, we might head south—that is, justify medical intervention by a capricious and confused combination of all three of the preceding justifications. That way—where the air is hazy and hot—paved with good medical intentions, lies hell. In such a system, the relations between sufferers and healers will be governed by the worst—the most despotic, capricious, and mendacious—elements of each of the three other systems. Patients, physicians, politicians, and people generally will then tend to fabricate increasingly arbitrary and self-serving definitions of illness and treatment and will try to impose them, by fraud and force, on anyone who resists. (The official acceptance of taking heroin as a disease and of being given methadone under medical auspices as a treatment is a signpost down that road; so is the official acceptance of personal disagreements as psychiatric diseases and of medically administered tortures as psychiatric treatments.)

I did not promise to offer, and did not offer, any solution to the problems exemplified by the situations cited. What I have offered, as I remarked at the beginning, is a map that I hope gives a reasonably accurate picture of the territory that all of us—whether as patients or doctors or both—must traverse in life. And I am offering one more thing—a reflection about it.

I know, or believe, that life is inherently tragic. In the Greek and Christian sense and tradition, tragedy is our fate. That is a given. But there is another kind of tragedy, the kind that we, as patients and physicians, as lawmakers and laymen, fabricate by evading the tragic choices thrust upon us by life. The belief that we can have a medico-ethical and medico-legal system that combines the virtues, but not the wickedness, of justifying medical interventions by illness, treatment, and consent is, I submit, such a tragedy. It is, in other words, not a tragic fate we must bear, but a tragic folly we must avoid.

# 4

# The Ethics of Addiction

Lest we take for granted that we know what drug addiction is, let us begin with some definitions.

According to the World Health Organization's Expert Committee on Drugs Liable to Produce Addiction,

> Drug addiction is a state of periodic or chronic intoxication detrimental to the individual and to society, produced by the repeated consumption of a drug (natural or synthetic). Its characteristics include: (1) an overpowering desire or need (compulsion) to continue taking the drug and to obtain it by any means, (2) a tendency to increase the dosage, and (3) a psychic (psychological) and sometimes physical dependence on the effects of the drug.[1]

Since this definition hinges on the harm done to the individual and to society by the consumption of the drug, it is clearly an ethical one. Moreover, by not specifying what is "detrimental" or who shall ascertain it and on what grounds, this definition immediately assimilates the problem of addiction with other psychiatric problems in which psychiatrists define the patient's dangerousness to himself and others. Actually, physicians regard as detrimental what people do to themselves but not what they do to people. For example, when college students smoke marijuana, that is detrimental; but when psychiatrists administer psychotropic drugs to involuntary mental patients, that is not detrimental.

1. Quoted in L. C. Kolb, *Noyes' Modern Clinical Psychiatry*, 7th ed. (Philadelphia: Saunders, 1968), p. 516.

The rest of the definition proposed by the World Health Organization is of even more dubious value. It speaks of an "overpowering desire" or "compulsion" to take the drug and of efforts to obtain it "by any means." Here again, we sink into the conceptual and semantic morass of psychiatric jargon. What is an "overpowering desire" if not simply a desire by which we choose to let ourselves be overpowered? And what is a "compulsion" if not simply an unresisted inclination to do something, and keep on doing it, even though someone thinks we should not be doing it?

Next, we come to the effort to obtain the addictive substance "by any means." That suggests that the substance is prohibited, or is very expensive for some other reason, and is hence difficult to obtain for the ordinary person rather than that the person who wants it has an inordinate craving for it. If there were an abundant and inexpensive supply of what the "addict" wants, there would be no reason for him to go to "any means" to obtain it. Does the World Health Organization's definition mean that one can be addicted only to a substance that is illegal or otherwise difficult to obtain? If so—and there is obviously some truth to the view that forbidden fruit tastes sweeter, although it cannot be denied that some things are sweet regardless of how the law treats them—then that surely removes the problem of addiction from the sphere of medicine and psychiatry and puts it squarely into that of morals and law.

The definition of addiction offered in *Webster's Third New International Dictionary of the English Language, Unabridged* exhibits the same difficulties. It defines addiction as "the compulsory uncontrolled use of habit-forming drugs beyond the period of medical need or under conditions harmful to society." This definition imputes lack of self-control to the addict over his taking or not taking a drug, a dubious proposition at best; at the same time, by qualifying an act as an addiction depending on whether or not it harms society, it offers a moral definition of an ostensibly medical condition.

Likewise, the currently popular term *drug abuse* places this behavior squarely in the category of ethics. For it is ethics that deals with the right and wrong uses of man's powers and possessions.

Clearly, drug addiction and drug abuse cannot be defined without specifying the proper and improper uses of certain pharmacologically active agents. The regular administration of morphine by a physician to a patient dying of cancer is the paradigm of the proper use of a narcotic, whereas even its occasional self-administration by a physically healthy person for the purpose of pharmacological pleasure is the paradigm of drug abuse.

I submit that these judgments have nothing whatever to do with medicine, pharmacology, or psychiatry. They are moral judgments. Indeed, our present views on addiction are astonishingly similar to some of our former views on sex. Intercourse in marriage with the aim of procreation used to be the paradigm of the proper use of one's sexual organs, whereas intercourse outside of marriage with the aim of carnal pleasure used to be the paradigm of their improper use. Until recently, masturbation—or self-abuse, as it was called—was professionally declared and popularly accepted as both the cause and the symptom of a variety of illnesses.[2]

To be sure, it is now virtually impossible to cite a contemporary American (or foreign) medical authority to support the concept of self-abuse. Medical opinion now holds that there is simply no such thing, that whether a person masturbates or not is medically irrelevant, and that engaging in the practice or refraining from it is a matter of personal morals or life-style. On the other hand, it is now virtually impossible to cite a contemporary American (or foreign) medical authority to oppose the concept of drug abuse. Medical opinion now holds that drug abuse is a major medical, psychiatric, and public-health problem; that drug addiction is a disease similar to diabetes, requiring prolonged (or lifelong) and carefully supervised medical treatment; and that taking or not taking drugs is primarily, if not solely, a matter of medical concern and responsibility.

Like any social policy, our drug laws may be examined from two entirely different points of view—technical and moral. Our present inclination is either to ignore the moral perspective or to mistake the technical for the moral.

An example of our misplaced overreliance on a technical ap-

2. See my *The Manufacture of Madness: A Comparative Study of the Inquisition and the Mental Health Movement* (New York: Harper & Row, 1970), pp. 180–206.

proach to the so-called drug problem is the professionalized mendacity about the dangerousness of certain types of drugs. Since most of the propagandists against drug abuse seek to justify certain repressive policies by appeals to the alleged dangerousness of various drugs, they often falsify the facts about the true pharmacological properties of the drugs they seek to prohibit. They do so for two reasons: first, because many substances in daily use are just as harmful as the substances they want to prohibit; second, because they realize that dangerousness alone is never a sufficiently persuasive argument to justify the prohibition of any drug, substance, or artifact. Accordingly, the more the "addiction-mongers" ignore the moral dimensions of the problem, the more they must escalate their fraudulent claims about the dangers of drugs.

To be sure, some drugs are more dangerous than others. It is easier to kill oneself with heroin than with aspirin. But it is also easier to kill oneself by jumping off a high building than a low one. In the case of drugs, we regard their potentiality for self-injury as justification for their prohibition; in the case of buildings, we do not.

Furthermore, we systematically blur and confuse the two quite different ways in which narcotics may cause death—by a deliberate act of suicide and by accidental overdosage.

As I have suggested elsewhere, we ought to consider suicide a basic human right.[3] If so, it is absurd to deprive an adult of a drug (or of anything else) because he might use it to kill himself. To do so is to treat everyone the way institutional psychiatrists treat the so-called suicidal mental patient: they not only imprison such a person but take everything away from him—shoelaces, belts, razor blades, eating utensils, and so forth—until the "patient" lies naked on a mattress in a padded cell, lest he kill himself. The result is the most degrading tyrannization in the annals of human history.

Death by accidental overdose is an altogether different matter. But can anyone doubt that this danger now looms so large precisely because the sale of narcotics and many other drugs is illegal? People who buy illicit drugs cannot be sure what drug they are getting or how much of it. Free trade in drugs, with governmental action limited to safeguarding the purity of the product and the veracity

3. See Chapter 6, "The Ethics of Suicide."

of the labeling, would reduce the risk of accidental overdose with "dangerous drugs" to the same levels that prevail, and that we find acceptable, with respect to other chemical agents and physical artifacts that abound in our complex technological society.

Although this essay is not intended as an exposition on the pharmacological properties of narcotics and other mind-affecting drugs, it might be well to say something more about the medical and social dangers they pose. Before proceeding to that task, I want to make clear, however, that in my view, regardless of their dangerousness, all drugs should be legalized (a misleading term I employ reluctantly as a concession to common usage). Although I recognize that some drugs—notably heroin, the amphetamines, and LSD among those now in vogue—may have undesirable personal or social consequences, I favor free trade in drugs for the same reason the Founding Fathers favored free trade in ideas: in an open society, it is none of the government's business what idea a man puts into his mind; likewise, it should be none of the government's business what drug he puts into his body.

It is a fundamental characteristic of human beings that they get used to things: one becomes habituated, or addicted, not only to narcotics, but to cigarettes, cocktails before dinner, orange juice for breakfast, comic strips, sex, and so forth. It is similarly a fundamental characteristic of living organisms that they acquire increasing tolerance to various chemical agents and physical stimuli: the first cigarette may cause nothing but nausea and headache; a year later, smoking three packs a day may be pure joy. Both alcohol and opiates are addictive, then, in the sense that the more regularly they are used, the more the user craves them and the greater his tolerance for them becomes. However, there is no mysterious process of "getting hooked" involved in any of this. It is simply an aspect of the universal biological propensity for learning, which is especially well-developed in man. The opiate habit, like the cigarette habit or the food habit, can be broken—usually without any medical assistance—provided the person wants to break it. Often he doesn't. And why indeed should he if he has nothing better to do with his life? Or as happens to be the case with morphine, if he can live an essentially normal life while under its influence? That, of course, sounds completely unbelievable, or worse—testimony to our "addiction" to half a century of systematic official mendacity about opiates, which we can break only by suffering the intellectual withdrawal symptoms that go with giving up treasured falsehoods.

Actually, opium is much less toxic than alcohol. Moreover, just as it is possible to be an alcoholic and work and be productive, so it is (or rather, it used to be) possible to be an opium addict and work and be productive. Thomas De Quincey and Samuel Taylor Coleridge were both opium takers, and "Kubla Khan," considered one of the most beautiful poems in the English language, was written while Coleridge was under the influence of opium.[4] According to a definitive study by Light and others published by the American Medical Association in 1929, "morphine addiction is not characterized by physical deterioration or impairment of physical fitness. . . . There is no evidence of change in the circulatory, hepatic, renal, or endocrine functions. When it is considered that these subjects had been addicted for at least five years, some of them as long as twenty years, these negative observations are highly significant."[5] In a 1928 study, Lawrence Kolb, an assistant surgeon general of the United States Public Health Service, found that of 119 persons addicted to opiates through medical practice, 90 had good industrial records and only 29 had poor ones:

> Judged by the output of labor and their own statements, none of the normal persons had their efficiency reduced by opium. Twenty-two of them worked regularly while taking opium for twenty-five years or more; one of them, a woman aged 81 and still alert mentally, had taken 3 grains of morphine daily for 65 years. [The usual therapeutic dose is ¼ grain, 3 to 4 grains being fatal for the nonaddict.] She gave birth to and raised six children, and managed her household affairs with more than average efficiency. A widow, aged 66, had taken 17 grains of morphine daily for most of 37 years. She is alert mentally . . . does physical labor every day, and makes her own living.[6]

4. A. Montagu, "The Long Search for Euphoria," *Reflections* 1 (May–June 1966): 65.

5. A. B. Light et al., *Opium Addiction* (Chicago: American Medical Association, 1929), p. 115; quoted in Alfred R. Lindesmith, *Addiction and Opiates* (Chicago: Aldine, 1968). p. 40.

6. L. Kolb, "Drug Addiction: A Study of Some Medical Cases," *Archives of Neurology and Psychiatry* 20 (1928): 178; quoted in Lindesmith, *Addiction and Opiates*, pp. 41–42.

I am not citing this evidence to recommend the opium habit. The point is that we must, in plain honesty, distinguish between pharmacological effects and personal inclinations. Some people take drugs to cope—to help them function and conform to social expectations. Others take them to cop out—to ritualize their refusal to function and conform to social expectations. Much of the drug abuse we now witness—perhaps nearly all of it—is of the second type. But instead of acknowledging that addicts are unable or unfit or unwilling to work and be normal, we prefer to believe that they act as they do because certain drugs—especially heroin, LSD, and the amphetamines—make them sick. If only we could get them well, so runs this comfortable and comforting view, they would become productive and useful citizens. To believe that is like believing that if an illiterate cigarette smoker would only stop smoking, he would become an Einstein. With a falsehood like that, one can go far. No wonder that politicians and psychiatrists love it.

The idea of free trade in drugs runs counter to another cherished notion of ours—namely, that everyone must work and that idleness is acceptable only under special conditions. In general, the obligation to work is greatest for healthy adult white males. We tolerate idleness on the part of children, women, blacks, the aged, and the sick, and we even accept the responsibility of supporting them. But the new wave of drug abuse affects mainly young adults, often white males who are, in principle at least, capable of working and supporting themselves. But they refuse: they drop out, adopting a life-style in which *not* working, *not* supporting oneself, *not* being useful to others, are positive values. These people challenge some of the most basic values of our society. It is hardly surprising, then, that society wants to retaliate, to strike back. Even though it would be cheaper to support addicts on welfare than to "treat" them, doing so would be legitimizing their life-style. That, "normal" society refuses to do. Instead, the majority acts as if it felt that, so long as it is going to spend its money on addicts, it is going to get something out of it. What society gets out of its war on addiction is what every persecutory movement provides for the persecutors: by defining a minority as evil (or sick), the majority confirms itself as good (or healthy). (If that can be done for the victim's own good, so much the better.) In short, the war on addiction is a part of that vast modern enterprise which I have named the "manufacture of madness." It is indeed a therapeutic enterprise, but with this grotesque twist: its beneficiaries are the therapists, and its victims are the patients.

Most of all perhaps, the idea of free trade in narcotics frightens people because they believe that vast masses of our population would spend their days and nights smoking opium or mainlining heroin instead of working and shouldering their responsibilities as citizens. But that is a bugaboo that does not deserve to be taken seriously. Habits of work and idleness are deep-seated cultural patterns; I doubt that free trade in drugs would convert industrious people from hustlers into hippies at the stroke of a legislative pen.

The other side of the economic coin regarding drugs and drug controls is actually far more important. The government is now spending millions of dollars—the hard-earned wages of hard-working Americans—to support a vast and astronomically expensive bureaucracy whose efforts not only drain our economic resources and damage our civil liberties but create ever more addicts and, indirectly, the crime associated with the traffic in illicit drugs. Although my argument about drug taking is moral and political and does not depend upon showing that free trade in drugs would also have fiscal advantages over our present policies, let me indicate briefly some of the economic aspects of the drug-control problem.

On April 1, 1967, New York State's narcotics addiction-control program, hailed as "the most massive ever tried in the nation," went into effect. "The program, which may cost up to $400 million in three years," reported *The New York Times,* "was hailed by Governor Rockefeller as 'the start of an unending war.' "[7] Three years later, it was conservatively estimated that the number of addicts in the state had tripled or quadrupled. New York State Senator John Hughes reported that the cost of caring for each addict during that time was $12,000 per year (as against $4,000 per year for patients in state mental hospitals).[8] It was a great time, though, for some of the ex-addicts themselves. In New York City's Addiction Services Agency, one ex-addict started at $6,500 a year

7. *The New York Times,* April 1, 1967.
8. Editorial, "About Narcotics," *Syracuse Herald-Journal*, March 6, 1969.

on November 27, 1967, and was making $16,000 seven months later. Another started at $6,500 on September 12, 1967, and went up to $18,100 by July 1, 1969.[9] The salaries of the medical bureaucrats in charge of the programs are similarly attractive. In short, the detection and rehabilitation of addicts is good business; and so was, in former days, the detection and rehabilitation of witches. We now know that the spread of witchcraft in the late Middle Ages was due more to the work of witchmongers than to the lure of witchcraft. Is it not possible that, similarly, the spread of addiction in our day is due more to the work of addictmongers than to the lure of narcotics?

Let us see how far some of the money spent on the war on addiction could go in supporting people who prefer to drop out of society and drug themselves. Their habit itself would, of course, cost next to nothing, for free trade would bring the price of narcotics down to a negligible amount. During the 1969–1970 fiscal year, the New York State Narcotics Addiction Control Commission had a budget of nearly $50 million, not including the budget for capital construction. Using that figure as a tentative base for calculation, here is what we come to: $100 million will support thirty thousand people at $3,300 per year; since the population of New York State is roughly one-tenth that of the nation, we arrive at a figure of $500 million to support one hundred and fifty thousand addicts nationally.

I am not advocating that we spend our hard-earned money in this way. I am only trying to show that free trade in narcotics would be more economical for those of us who work, even if we had to support legions of addicts, than is our present program of trying to "cure" them. Moveover, I have not even made use, in my economic estimates, of the incalculable sums we would thus save by reducing crimes now engendered by the illegal traffic in drugs.

Clearly, the argument that marijuana—or heroin, or methadone, or morphine—is prohibited because it is addictive or dangerous cannot be supported by facts. For one thing, there are many drugs —from insulin to penicillin—that are neither addictive nor danger-

9. *The New York Times,* June 29, 1970.

ous but are nevertheless also prohibited—they can be obtained only through a physician's prescription. For another, there are many things—from dynamite to guns—that are much more dangerous than narcotics (especially to others) but are not prohibited. As everyone knows, it is still possible in the United States to walk into a store and walk out with a shotgun. We enjoy that right not because we do not believe that guns are dangerous, but because we believe even more strongly that civil liberties are precious. At the same time, it is not possible in the United States to walk into a store and walk out with a bottle of barbiturates, codeine, or other drugs. We are now deprived of that right because we have come to value medical paternalism more highly than the right to obtain and use drugs without recourse to medical intermediaries.

I submit, therefore, that our so-called drug-abuse problem is an integral part of our present social ethic, which accepts "protections" and repressions justified by appeals to health similar to those that medieval societies accepted when they were justified by appeals to faith.[10] Drug abuse (as we now know it) is one of the inevitable consequences of the medical monopoly over drugs—a monopoly whose value is daily acclaimed by science and law, state and church, the professions and the laity. As the Church formerly regulated man's relations to God, so Medicine now regulates his relations to his body. Deviation from the rules set forth by the Church was then considered to be heresy and was punished by appropriate theological sanctions, called *penance*; deviation from the rules set forth by Medicine is now considered to be drug abuse (or some sort of mental illness) and is punished by appropriate medical sanctions, called *treatment*.

The problem of drug abuse will thus be with us so long as we live under medical tutelage. This is not to say that if all access to drugs were free, some people would not medicate themselves in ways that might upset us or harm them. That of course is precisely what happened when religious practices became free.

What I am suggesting is that although addiction is ostensibly a medical and pharmacological problem, actually it is a moral and

10. See my *Ideology and Insanity: Essays on the Psychiatric Dehumanization of Man* (Garden City, N.Y.: Doubleday, Anchor Press, 1970).

political problem. We talk as if we were trying to ascertain which drugs *are* toxic, but we act as if we were trying to decide which drugs *ought to be* prohibited.

We ought to know, however, that there is no necessary connection between facts and values, between what is and what ought to be. Thus, objectively quite harmful acts, objects, or persons may be accepted and tolerated—by minimizing their dangerousness. Conversely, objectively quite harmless acts, objects, or persons may be prohibited and persecuted—by exaggerating their dangerousness. It is always necessary to distinguish—and especially so when dealing with social policy—between description and prescription, fact and rhetoric, truth and falsehood.

To command adherence, social policy must be respected; and to be respected, it must be considered legitimate. In our society, there are two principal methods of legitimizing policy—social tradition and scientific judgment. More than anything else, time is the supreme ethical arbiter. Whatever a social practice might be, if people engage in it generation after generation, then that practice becomes acceptable.

Many opponents of illegal drugs admit that nicotine may be more harmful to health than marijuana; nevertheless, they argue that smoking cigarettes should be legal but smoking marijuana should not be, because the former habit is socially accepted while the latter is not. That is a perfectly reasonable argument. But let us understand it for what it is—a plea for legitimizing old and accepted practices and illegitimizing novel and unaccepted ones. It is a justification that rests on precedence, not on evidence.

The other method of legitimizing policy, increasingly more important in the modern world, is through the authority of science. In matters of health, a vast and increasingly elastic category, physicians thus play important roles as legitimizers and illegitimizers. One result is that, regardless of the pharmacological effects of a drug on the person who takes it, if he obtains it through a physician and uses it under medical supervision, that use is, ipso facto, legitimate and proper; but if he obtains it through nonmedical channels and uses it without medical supervision (and especially if the drug is illegal and the individual uses it solely for the purpose of altering his mental state), then that use is, ipso facto, illegitimate and improper. In short, being medicated by a doctor is drug use, while self-medication (especially with certain classes of drugs) is drug abuse.

That too is a perfectly reasonable arrangement. But let us understand it for what it is—a plea for legitimizing what doctors do, because they do it with good, therapeutic intent; and for illegitimizing what laymen do, because they do it with bad, self-abusive (masturbatory) intent. It is a justification that rests on the principles of professionalism, not of pharmacology. That is why we applaud the systematic medical use of methadone and call it "treatment for heroin addiction," but decry the occasional nonmedical use of marijuana and call it "dangerous drug abuse."

Our present concept of drug abuse thus articulates and symbolizes a fundamental policy of scientific medicine—namely, that a layman should not medicate his own body but should place its medical care under the supervision of a duly accredited physician. Before the Reformation, the practice of true Christianity rested on a similar policy—namely, that a layman should not himself commune with God but should place his spiritual care under the supervision of a duly accredited priest. The self-interests of the Church and of Medicine in such policies are obvious enough. What might be less obvious is the interest of the laity in them: by delegating responsibility for the spiritual and medical welfare of the people to a class of authoritatively accredited specialists, those policies—and the practices they ensure—relieve individuals from assuming the burdens of those responsibilities for themselves. As I see it, our present problems with drug use and drug abuse are just one of the consequences of our pervasive ambivalence about personal autonomy and responsibility.

Luther's chief heresy was to remove the priest as intermediary between man and God, giving the former direct access to the latter. He also demystified the language in which man could henceforth address God, approving for that purpose what until then had significantly been called the *vulgar tongue*. Perhaps it is true that familiarity breeds contempt: Protestantism was not just a new form of Christianity, but the beginning of its end, at least as it had been known until then.

I propose a medical reformation analogous to the Protestant Reformation—specifically, a "protest" against the systematic mystification of man's relationship to his body and his professionalized separation from it. The immediate aim of the reform would be to remove the physician as intermediary between man and his body and to give the layman direct access to the language and contents of the pharmacopoeia. It is significant that until recently physicians wrote prescriptions in Latin and that medical diagnoses and treatments are still couched in a jargon whose chief aim is to awe and mystify the laity. If man had unencumbered access to his own body and the means of chemically altering it, it would spell the end of Medicine, at least as we now know it. That is why, with faith in Medicine so strong, there is little interest in this kind of medical reform: physicians fear the loss of their privileges; laymen, the loss of their protections.

Our present policies with respect to drug use and drug abuse thus constitute a covert plea for legitimizing certain privileges on the part of physicians and illegitimizing certain practices on the part of everyone else. The upshot is that we act as if we believed that only doctors should be allowed to dispense narcotics, just as we used to believe that only priests should be allowed to dispense holy water.

Finally, since luckily we still do not live in the utopian perfection of one world, our technical approach to the drug problem has led, and will undoubtedly continue to lead, to some curious attempts to combat it.

In one such attempt, the American government succeeded in pressuring Turkey to restrict its farmers from growing poppy (the source of opium, morphine, and heroin).[11] If turnabout is fair play, perhaps we should expect the Turkish government to pressure the United States to restrict its farmers from growing barley. Or should we assume that Muslims have enough self-control to leave alcohol alone but Christians need all the controls politicians, policemen, and physicians, both native and foreign, can bring to bear on them to enable them to leave opiates alone?

11. "Pursuit of the Poppy," *Time*, September 14, 1970, p. 28.

In another such attempt, the California Civil Liberties Union sued to enforce a paroled heroin addict's "right to methadone maintenance treatment."[12] In this view, the addict has more rights than the nonaddict: for the former, methadone, supplied at the taxpayer's expense, is a right; for the latter, methadone, supplied at his own expense, is evidence of addiction to it.

I believe that just as we regard freedom of speech and religion as fundamental rights, so we should also regard freedom of self-medication as a fundamental right; and that instead of mendaciously opposing or mindlessly promoting illicit drugs, we should, paraphrasing Voltaire, make this maxim our rule: I disapprove of what you take, but I will defend to the death your right to take it!

To be sure, like most rights, the right of self-medication should apply only to adults; and it should not be an unqualified right. Since these are important qualifications, it is necessary to specify their precise range.

John Stuart Mill said (approximately) that a person's right to swing his arm ends where his neighbor's nose begins. Similarly, the limiting condition with respect to self-medication should be the inflicting of actual (as against symbolic) harm on others.

Our present practices with respect to alcohol embody and reflect this individualistic ethic. We have the right to buy, possess, and consume alcoholic beverages. Regardless of how offensive drunkenness might be to a person, he cannot interfere with another person's right to become inebriated so long as that person drinks in the privacy of his own home or at some other appropriate location and so long as he conducts himself in an otherwise law-abiding manner. In short, we have a right to be intoxicated—in private. Public intoxication is considered to be an offense against others and is therefore a violation of the criminal law.

The same principle applies to sexual conduct. Sexual intercourse, especially between husband and wife, is surely a right. But it is a right that must be exercised at home or at some other appropriate location; it is not a right in a public park or on a downtown street.

12. "CLU Says Addict Has Right to Use Methadone," *Civil Liberties*, July 1970, p. 5.

It makes sense that what is a right in one place may become, by virtue of its disruptive or disturbing effect on others, an offense somewhere else.

The right to self-medication should be hedged in by similar limits. Public intoxication, not only with alcohol but with any drug, should be an offense punishable by the criminal law. Furthermore, acts that may injure others—such as driving a car—should, when carried out in a drug-intoxicated state, be punished especially strictly and severely. The habitual use of certain drugs, such as alcohol and opiates, may also harm others indirectly by rendering the subject unmotivated for working and thus unemployed. In a society that supports the unemployed, such a person would, as a consequence of his own conduct, place a burden on the shoulders of his working neighbors. How society might best guard itself against that sort of hazard I cannot discuss here. However, it is obvious that prohibiting the use of habit-forming drugs offers no protection against that risk, but only adds to the tax burdens laid upon the productive members of society.

The right to self-medication must thus entail unqualified responsibility for the effects of one's drug-intoxicated behavior on others. For unless we are willing to hold ourselves responsible for our own behavior and hold others responsible for theirs, the liberty to ingest or inject drugs degenerates into a license to injure others. But here is the catch: we are exceedingly reluctant to hold people responsible for their misbehavior. That is why we prefer diminishing rights to increasing responsibilities. The former requires only the passing of laws, which can then be more or less freely violated or circumvented; whereas the latter requires prosecuting and punishing offenders, which can be accomplished only by just laws justly enforced. The upshot is that we increasingly substitute tender-hearted tyranny for tough-spirited liberty.

Such then would be the situation of adults were we to regard the freedom to take drugs as a fundamental right similar to the freedom to read and to worship. What would be the situation of children? Since many people who are now said to be drug addicts or drug abusers are minors, it is especially important that we think clearly about this aspect of the problem.

I do not believe, and I do not advocate, that children should have a right to ingest, inject, or otherwise use any drug or substance they want. Children do not have the right to drive, drink, vote, marry, or make binding contracts. They acquire those rights at various ages, coming into their full possession at maturity, usually between the ages of eighteen and twenty-one. The right to self-medication should similarly be withheld until maturity.

In this connection, it is well to remember that children lack even such basic freedoms as the opportunity to read what they wish or worship God as they choose, freedoms we consider elementary rights for adult Americans. In those as well as other important respects, children are wholly under the jurisdiction of their parents or guardians. The disastrous fact that many parents fail to exercise proper authority over the conduct of their children does not, in my opinion, justify depriving adults of the right to engage in conduct we deem undesirable for children. That remedy only further aggravates the situation. For if we consider it proper to prohibit the use of narcotics by adults to prevent their abuse by children, then we would have to consider it proper also to prohibit sexual intercourse, driving automobiles, piloting airplanes—indeed virtually everything!—because those activities too are likely to be abused by children.

In short, I suggest that "dangerous" drugs be treated more or less as alcohol and tobacco are treated now. (That does not mean that I believe the state should make their use a source of tax revenue.) Neither the use of narcotics nor their possession should be prohibited, but only their sale to minors. Of course, that would result in the ready availability of all kinds of drugs among minors—though perhaps their availability would be no greater than it is now but only more visible and hence more easily subject to proper controls. That arrangement would place responsibility for the use of all drugs by children where it belongs: on parents and their children. That is where the major responsibility rests for the use of alcohol and tobacco. It is a tragic symptom of our refusal to take personal liberty and responsibility seriously that there appears to be no public desire to assume a similar stance toward other dangerous drugs.

Consider what would happen should a child bring a bottle of gin to school and get drunk there. Would the school authorities blame the local liquor stores as pushers? Or would they blame the parents and the child himself? There is liquor in practically every home in America and yet children rarely bring liquor to school, whereas marijuana, LSD, and heroin—substances that children do not find in the home and whose very possession is a criminal offense—frequently find their way into the school.

Our attitude toward sexual activity provides another model for our attitude toward drugs. Although we generally discourage children below a certain age from engaging in sexual activities with others (we no longer "guard" them against masturbation), we do not prohibit such activities by law. What we do prohibit by law is the sexual seduction of children by adults. The pharmacological seduction of children by adults should be similarly punishable. In other words, adults who give or sell drugs to children should be regarded as offenders. Such a specific and limited prohibition—contrasted with the kind of generalized prohibitions that we had under the Volstead Act or have now against countless drugs—would be relatively easy to enforce. Moreover, it would probably be rarely violated, for there would be little psychological interest and no economic profit in doing so. On the other hand, the use of drugs by and among children (without the direct participation of adults) should be a matter entirely outside the scope of the criminal law, just as is their engaging in sexual activities under like circumstances.

There is of course a fatal flaw in my proposal. Its adoption would remove minors from the ranks of our most cherished victims: we could no longer spy on them and persecute them in the name of protecting them from committing drug abuse on themselves—a practice we have substituted for our spying on them and persecuting them in order to protect them from committing self-abuse on themselves (that is, masturbating).[13] Hence, we cannot, and indeed we shall not, abandon such therapeutic tyrannization and treat children as young persons entitled to dignity from us and owing responsibility to us until we are ready to cease psychiatrically oppressing children—"in their own best interests."

13. See *The Manufacture of Madness*, chap. 11.

Sooner or later, we shall have to confront the basic moral dilemma underlying our drug problem: does a person have the right to take a drug—any drug—not because he needs it to cure an illness, but because he wants to take it?

The Declaration of Independence speaks of our inalienable right to "life, liberty, and the pursuit of happiness." How are we to interpret that phrase? By asserting that we ought to be free to pursue happiness by playing golf or watching television but not by drinking alcohol, or smoking marijuana, or ingesting amphetamines?

The Constitution and the Bill of Rights are silent on the subject of drugs. Their silence would seem to imply that the adult citizen has, or ought to have, the right to medicate his own body as he sees fit. Were that not the case, why should there have been a need for a constitutional amendment to outlaw drinking? But if ingesting alcohol was, and is now again, a constitutional right, is ingesting opium, or heroin, or barbiturates, or anything else not also such a right? If it is, then the Harrison Narcotic Act is not only a bad law but unconstitutional as well, because it prescribes in a legislative act what ought to be promulgated in a constitutional amendment.

The nagging questions remain. As American citizens, do we and should we have the right to take narcotics or other drugs? Further, if we take drugs and conduct ourselves as responsible and law-abiding citizens, do we and should we have a right to remain unmolested by the government? Lastly, if we take drugs and break the law, do we and should we have a right to be treated as persons accused of a crime rather than as patients accused of being mentally ill?

These are fundamental questions that are conspicuous by their absence from all contemporary discussions of problems of drug addiction and drug abuse. In this area as in so many others, we have allowed a moral problem to be disguised as a medical question and have then engaged in shadowboxing with metaphorical diseases and medical attempts, ranging from the absurd to the appalling, to combat them.

The result is that instead of debating the use of drugs in moral and political terms, we define our task as the ostensibly narrow technical problem of protecting people from poisoning themselves with substances for whose use they cannot possibly assume responsibility. That, I think, best explains the frightening national consensus against personal responsibility for taking drugs and for one's conduct while under their influence. In 1965, for example, when President Johnson sought a bill imposing tight federal controls over "pep pills" and "goof balls," the bill cleared the House by a unanimous vote, 402 to 0.

The failure of such measures to curb the "drug menace" has served only to inflame our legislators' enthusiasm for them. In October 1970, the Senate passed, again by a unanimous vote (54 to 0), "a major narcotics crackdown bill hailed as a keystone in President Nixon's anticrime program. Added to the bill were strong new measures for the treatment and rehabilitation of drug abusers."[14] In December 1971, the Senate approved—this time by a unanimous vote of 92 to 0—a "$1 billion-plus bill to mount the nation's first all-out, coordinated attack on the insidious menace of drug abuse";[15] in February 1972, the House voted 380 to 0 for a $411 million, three-year program to combat drug abuse; and in March, the House voted 366 to 0, to authorize a $1 billion three-year federal attack on drug abuse.

To me, such unremitting unanimity on this issue can mean one thing only: an evasion of the actual problem and an attempt to master it by attacking and overpowering a scapegoat—"dangerous drugs" and "drug abusers." There is an ominous resemblance between the unanimity with which all "reasonable" men—especially politicians, physicians, and priests—formerly supported the protective measures of society against witches and Jews and now support them against drug addicts and drug abusers.

Finally, those repeated unanimous votes on far-reaching measures to combat drug abuse are bitter reminders that when the chips are really down, that is, when democratic lawmakers can preserve their intellectual and moral integrity only by going against certain popular myths, they prove to be either mindless or spineless. They prefer running with the herd to courting unpopularity and risking reelection.

14. *Syracuse Post-Standard*, October 8, 1970.
15. *The International Herald Tribune*, December 4–5, 1971.

After all is said and done—after millions of words are written, thousands of laws are enacted, and countless numbers of people are "treated" for "drug abuse"—it all comes down to whether we accept or reject the ethical principle John Stuart Mill so clearly enunciated in 1859:

> The only purpose for which power can be rightfully exercised over any member of a civilized community, against his will, is to prevent harm to others. His own good, either physical or moral, is not a sufficient warrant. He cannot rightfully be compelled to do or forebear because it will make him happier, because, in the opinions of others, to do so would be wise, or even right. . . . In the part [of his conduct] which merely concerns himself, his independence is, of right, absolute. Over himself, over his own body and mind, the individual is sovereign.[16]

The basic issue underlying the problem of addiction—and many other problems, such as sexual activity between consenting adults, pornography, contraception, gambling, and suicide—is simple but vexing: in a conflict between the individual and the state, where should the former's autonomy end and the latter's right to intervene begin?

One way out of the dilemma lies through concealment: by disguising the moral and political question as a medical and therapeutic problem, we can, to protect the physical and mental health of patients, exalt the state, oppress the individual, and claim benefits for both.

The other way out of it lies through confrontation: by recognizing the problem for what it is, we can choose to maximize the sphere of action of the state at the expense of the individual or of the individual at the expense of the state. In other words, we can commit ourselves to the view that the state, the representative of many, is more important than the individual and that it therefore has the right, indeed the duty, to regulate the life of the individual in the best interests of the group. Or we can commit ourselves to the view that individual dignity and liberty are the supreme values of life and that the foremost duty of the state is to protect and promote those values.

In short, we must choose between the ethic of collectivism and the ethic of individualism and pay the price of either—or of both.

16. J. S. Mill, *On Liberty* (Chicago: Regnery, 1955), p. 13.

# 5

# The Ethics of Behavior Therapy

My aim in this essay is to offer an exposition of the moral dimensions of behavior therapy; to identify the actual activities of behavior therapists; and to indicate my acceptance of some of their interventions, my rejection of others, and the justifications for my judgments.

Let me begin by registering my agreement with the contention of behavior therapists that, like all therapists, they influence behavior. My unqualified agreement with behavior therapists ends right here. Although there are qualified agreements between us on some other points—such as the significance of actual behavior rather than its verbal rationalization or the importance of classifying the patient's and professional's goals in therapy—my position is divided from theirs (as it is from that of most other psychiatrists and psychotherapists): I insist on distinguishing sharply between voluntary and involuntary psychotherapeutic interventions, between choice leading to contract and coercion leading to capitulation—in short, between doing something *for* a person and doing something *to* him.

I can sense that at this point many behavior therapists will want to interrupt and declare their own allegiance—no doubt sincere—to the principle of informed consent to treatment and their opposition—no doubt well meant—to the use of psychiatric or psychological technology for punishment. Such protests, I am afraid, leave me as unconvinced and unmoved as do the similar protests of the training analysts and institutional psychiatrists that they labor always and only for the benefit of their analysands or patients. It is an old saying that words are cheap, a maxim with which behavior therapists can hardly quarrel. It is therefore not very important or interesting what behavior therapists *say* about what they do or why they do it; what is important and interesting is what they *do* and how they describe it. So examined, much of what they do appears to be plainly coercive, imposed on the client or patient by force or fraud.

Before illustrating this contention, let me anticipate and try to rebut an objection that may be raised here. "There are many behavior therapists who do many things," so the objection might run. "While it may be true that among all these interventions there are some that are coerced or involuntary, they represent a small fraction of the total, and hence they are not representative of what behavior therapy *really* is."

That sort of argument is, in my opinion, disingenuous. Although I do not know, and I dare say no one does, what the exact proportion of voluntary to involuntary behavior-therapeutic interventions is—whether it is 99 to 1, or 1 to 1, or 1 to 99—one thing is clear from a perusal of the published literature in the field: behavior therapy is used routinely on patients who do not or cannot give informed consent to it.

Modern behavior therapy is tainted, it seems to me, with a hereditary defect that it has acquired from the mother out of whose womb it emerged. I refer to the social context in which behavior therapy was first carried out: the state mental hospital.

The experiments in question are those performed by Ogden Lindsley and B. F. Skinner at the Metropolitan State Hospital in Waltham, Massachusetts, under the auspices of the Department of Psychiatry at Harvard Medical School, supported by grants from the Office of Naval Research and the Rockefeller Foundation, and reported in 1954. Lindsley and Skinner studied fifteen male patients who had been hospitalized for an average of seventeen years. Their conclusions are best stated in their own words:

> The similarity between the performance of psychotic patients and the performance of "normal" rats, pigeons, and dogs on two schedules of intermittent reinforcement suggests that psychotic behavior is controlled to some extent by the reinforcing properties of the immediate

physical environment, and that the effects of different schedules of reinforcement upon the behavior of psychotics should be investigated further.[1]

There is no need to encumber this presentation with my objections to Skinner's ideas and ethics, as I have set them forth elsewhere;[2] suffice it to note that in the above passage Lindsley and Skinner put the word *normal*, with which they qualify rats, in quotation marks but do not put the word *psychotic*, with which they qualify persons, in quotation marks. In other words, they accept as obvious that just as some individuals are diabetic or leukemic, so others are psychotic. I consider that a fatal flaw to everything that follows in Skinner's work having to do with "mental patients," as well as in the work of behavior therapists who accept that psychiatric premise.[3] Finally, that Lindsley and Skinner here also accept—and that all those who have subsequently referred to this work approvingly also accept—the moral legitimacy of incarcerating "psychotics" and then "treating" them against their will is obvious. That this carries with it an ethical burden that invalidates all subsequent work based on this model may be less obvious but is, I think, the case.

During the past several decades, a great deal of behavior therapy has been conducted in closed institutions—that is, in mental hospitals and prisons. As I mentioned earlier, I do not know, and I doubt if anyone does, whether more behavior therapy is conducted coercively than contractually. The fact remains that many of the recipients of the "benefits" of behavior therapy have been, and continue to be, persons whose status as clients or patients was, *pro forma* or de facto, involuntary. I shall comment first on behavior therapy in mental hospitals and then on behavior therapy in prisons.

Lindsley's detailed report on the experiments to which I referred

1. O. R. Lindsley and B. F. Skinner, "A Method for the Experimental Analysis of the Behavior of Psychotic Patients," *American Psychologist* 9 (August 1954): 419.

2. See my review of *About Behavior* by B. F. Skinner, *Libertarian Review* 3 (December 1974): 6–7.

3. See my *The Myth of Mental Illness: Foundations of a Theory of Personal Conduct*, rev. ed. (New York: Harper & Row, 1974).

already seems to set the tone for much of this sort of work. "The free operant method," he writes in 1956, "can be used, with very little modification, to measure the behavior of any animal from a turtle to a normal genius." It is odd that Lindsley here qualifies genius as "normal" because in the very next sentence he proposes to apply this method to "psychotics": "Since neither instructions nor rapport with the experimenter are demanded, the method is particularly appropriate in analyzing the behavior of non-verbal, lowly motivated, chronic psychotic patients."[4]

The patients reported on in the study had been incarcerated for an average of twelve years. Here briefly is what Lindsley says about them and what he did with them:

> We selected patients who were preferably not on parole, not working in hospital industries, not receiving active therapy, not receiving visitors, and not going on home visits. We did this in order to minimize extraneous variables and to facilitate patient handling. . . . Our standard procedure is to go up to a patient, for the first time, on the ward and ask him if he wants to come with us and get some candy or cigarettes. Those who do not answer are led, if they do not follow us, to the laboratory. If at any time a patient balks or refuses, he is left on the ward.[5]

Evidently, Lindsley believes that dealing with the patients in that way is enough to establish that they are not coerced. He completely ignores the fact that he is functioning as a member of the authority structure of the hospital. I consider such work to be only slightly less odious than experimenting on the inmates of concentration camps. I say that because I believe it is the moral duty of psychologists and psychiatrists to safeguard the dignity and liberty of people generally, and, in particular, of those with whom they work. If instead they take professional advantage of the imprisoned status of incarcerated individuals or populations, they are, in my opinion, criminals.

Much of the literature on the use of behavior therapy in mental institutions exudes a similarly offensive moral odor. A few illustrations must suffice.

4. O. R. Lindsley, "Operant Conditioning Methods Applied to Research in Chronic Schizophrenia," *Psychiatric Research Reports* 5 (1956): 118–119.
5. Ibid., p. 128.

A paper by Isaacs, Thomas, and Goldiamond entitled "Application of Operant Conditioning to Reinstate Verbal Behavior in Psychotics" is typical. The title itself is deceptive, as it is a scientistic way of describing an effort to make nontalkative people talk. This is the authors' description of their first patient:

> Patient A—The S [subject] was brought to a group therapy session with other chronic schizophrenics (who were verbal), but he sat in the position in which he was placed and continued the withdrawal behaviors which characterized him. He remained impassive and stared ahead even when cigarettes, which other members accepted, were offered to him and were waved before his face.[6]

There is no evidence that the investigators made any effort to discover what the patient wanted and to satisfy his desires. The idea that this man, who preferred not to talk, should talk was clearly the investigators', which they then imposed on him by trying to bribe him with cigarettes. This subject, as well as the other one mentioned in this paper, was, moreover, an involuntary mental patient: "Patient A, classified as a catatonic schizophrenic, 40, became completely mute almost immediately upon commitment 19 years ago."[7] Perhaps he did not like the company he was condemned to keep.

Although the authors relate with evident professional pride how they tried to make the man talk by offering him cigarettes (whose "abuse" is now about to be declared a newly discovered form of mental illness by the American Psychiatric Association), there is no evidence that they tried to achieve the same result by freeing him from psychiatric imprisonment.

The *use*—and I am setting this term in italics to call attention to it—of helpless, incarcerated, so-called schizophrenic patients as subjects for behavior therapy is, of course, a routine matter. I could fill hundreds of pages with excerpts from papers reporting on such treatments. Here is a typical report by Teodoro Aylion, a prominent behavior therapist: "The subjects were two female patients in a mental hospital. Both patients had been classified as

6. W. Isaacs, J. Thomas, and I. Goldiamond, "Application of Operant Conditioning to Reinstate Verbal Behavior in Psychotics," in L. P. Ullmann and L. Krasner, eds., *Case Studies in Behavior Modification* (New York: Holt, Rinehart & Winston, 1965), p. 69.

7. Ibid.

schizophrenic. . . . Anne was 54 years old and had been in the hospital for 20 years. Emelda was 60 years old and had been in the hospital for 18 years."[8]

Anne and Emelda would not eat unless fed, and the purpose of Ayllon's treatment was to make them feed themselves. The beneficiaries of this sort of treatment are clear enough. Whether a therapist should be proud or ashamed to do this sort of thing is just the kind of question evaded by single-minded attention to the technical aspects of behavior (or other) therapy.

In another paper Ayllon makes it even clearer that, regardless of his professed aim, what he actually does is to make "difficult" patients easier to manage:

> The patient was a 47-year-old female diagnosed as a chronic schizophrenic . . . hospitalized for 9 years. Upon studying the patient's behavior on the ward, it became apparent that the nursing staff spent considerable time caring for her. In particular, there were three aspects of her behavior which seemed to defy solution. The first was stealing food. The second was the hoarding of the ward's towels in her room. The third undesirable aspect of her behavior consisted in her wearing excessive clothing, e.g., half-dozen dresses, several pairs of stockings, sweaters, and so on.[9]

Ayllon devised a complicated social ritual to deal with the food stealing that, in his own words, "resulted in the patient missing a meal whenever she attempted to steal food."[10] In plain English, for stealing food the patient was punished by starvation.

In view of the support that behavior therapy and behavior therapists lend to the principles and practices of institutional psychiatry, it is not surprising that the American Psychiatric Association's Task Force on Behavior Therapy has issued a glowing report on it. The following excerpts from the report reveal the close ties between coercive psychiatry and the conditioning therapies:

8. T. Ayllon, "Some Behavioral Problems Associated with Eating in Chronic Schizophrenic Patients," in Ullmann and Krasner, eds., *Case Studies*, pp. 73–74.

9. T. Ayllon, "Intensive Treatment of Psychotic Behavior by Stimulus Satiation and Food Reinforcement," in Ullmann and Krasner, eds., *Case Studies*, p. 78.

10. Ibid., p. 79.

> The early development of the token economy system took place almost exclusively within the context of the closed ward psychiatric treatment center and was found quite useful in preventing or overcoming the habit deterioration or social breakdown syndrome that accompanies prolonged custodial hospitalization, whatever the initial diagnosis.[11]

Assuming its typical posture—foot in mouth—the American Psychiatric Association here spills the beans: behavior therapy is useful because it enables psychiatric wardens to impose "prolonged custodial hospitalization" on their victims, while sparing them the unpleasantness of having to put up with the victims' "habit deterioration."

The task force's remarks on the abuses of behavior therapy incriminate this form of intervention still further. Here too the American Psychiatric Association persists in its habitual rhetoric in trying to justify the psychiatric oppression of patients:

> Therapists must be on guard against requests for treatment that take the form "Make him 'behave,' " in which the intention of the request is to make the person conform. . . . One safeguard against this is to obtain the patient's informed agreement about the goals and methods of the therapy program whenever possible.[12]

Whenever possible! And when not possible, then of course it is permissible to impose behavior therapy without consent.

The American Psychiatric Association's hypocrisy concerning coercion is further amplified in the task force's remarks about aversive therapies:

> First, aversive methods should be carried out under the surveillance of the therapist's clinical peers and colleagues; second, aversive methods especially should be used only with the patient's informed consent. . . . If the therapist is aware of precisely what reinforces his own behavior, he can avoid exploitation in his work with patients.[13]

This declaration about limiting the use of aversive therapies to consenting clients is hypocritical. If that is what the writers of this

11. American Psychiatric Association, Task Force on Behavior Therapy, *Behavior Therapy in Psychiatry* (New York: Aronson, 1974), p. 25.

12. Ibid., p. 100.

13. Ibid., p. 102.

report and the American Psychiatric Association itself believe, why have they not demanded the criminal prosecution of those who use aversive therapy on involuntary clients or patients—for example, the psychiatrists and psychologists at the California Medical Facility in Vacaville, where succinylcholine was used as an "aversive tool" and where this "therapy" was imposed on at least five inmates whose consent was solicited but not obtained?[14] Since these inmates were asked for consent, the "therapists" must have considered them capable of giving consent. The fact that the professionals treated them without it—in the face of the inmates' explicit refusal to give consent—establishes, in my mind at least, that the therapists acted criminally. The silence of behavior modifiers about such uses of their ideas and interventions renders their pious pronouncements about consent and contract less than persuasive.

In this connection, I should like to call attention to an important paper by Dougal Mackay in which he demonstrates the utter incompatibility between the basic principles of behavior therapy and the imagery and ideology of psychiatry, which behavior therapists nevertheless enthusiastically support.[15] Why they do so is, of course, clear enough. Deprived of the professional support of medicine and the social justification of treatment, behavior therapists would have to sell their services in the open market; there they could not coerce involuntary clients to do things they did not want to do, and they could not con the public and the state into supporting them at the taxpayers' expense. That would put them back where the psychoanalysts were in Vienna in 1900—which is exactly where they belong.

The use of behavior therapy in prisons, especially when its results influence the judgments of the prison personnel and parole boards,

14. T. S. Szasz, ed., *The Age of Madness: The History of Involuntary Mental Hospitalization Presented in Selected Texts* (Garden City, N.Y.: Doubleday, Anchor Press, 1973), pp. 356–359.

15. D. Mackay, "Behavior Modification and Its Psychiatric Straitjacket," *New Behaviour*, May 15, 1975, pp. 153–157. In this connection, see also D. A. Begelman, "Ethical and Legal Issues in Behavior Modification," in M. Hersen, R. Eisler, and P. Miller, eds., *Progress in Behavior Modification* (New York: Academic Press, 1975), vol. 1, pp. 159–189; and G. C. Davison and R. B. Stuart, "Behavior Therapy and Civil Liberties," *American Psychologist* 30 (July 1975): 755–763.

raises fundamental questions, not only about infringements on the prisoners' rights, but also about the nature and limits of the penal system. In the United States, it would be clearly unconstitutional to demand as a condition of release from prison that a prisoner convert from religion A to religion B. Evidently, it is not unconstitutional to demand that he convert from behavior A to behavior B, especially when the conversion is called behavior therapy.

Jonathan Cole, a prominent apologist for institutional psychiatry, offers this view about the use of behavior therapy in prisons:

> Assuming a prisoner is clearly informed about the nature of a behavior modification program and has the option to withdraw from it if he finds it unpleasant or undesirable, there seems to be no conceivable objection to offering a prisoner or a group of prisoners a chance to change behaviors which they agree need changing.[16]

Cole finds it inconceivable that anyone should object to such an arrangement because of the possibilities of abuse inherent in it, and he offers no remedy for prison authorities' or parole-board members' punishing prisoners for refusing such "offers"—in fact, he does not even consider that possibility. Yet it seems real enough, as the following example shows:

> Three convicted child molesters have sued to end a state program which uses electric shock and social conditioning to change their sex behavior. The three inmates say the program is unconstitutional because they are allegedly forced to participate to gain parole. As part of the program's therapy, shock is administered to the groin during a slide show of nude children. The shock stops when slides of nude women are shown.[17]

Showing slides of nude women to male prisoners and calling it therapy is imaginative indeed. But why not display live models? Better still, why not supply the prisoners with prostitutes? Perhaps I should make it clear that I advance these suggestions tongue in cheek. Such a caveat is necessary, as pimps and procurers with

16. J. O. Cole, "What's in a Word? Or Guilt by Definition, Part II," *Medical Tribune*, June 18, 1975, p. 9.

17. *New York Post*, January 30, 1975.

medical credentials now claim to be, and are widely accepted as, therapists.

Behavior therapy has long been an integral part of the program at the Patuxent Institution, a hybrid between a prison and a mental hospital and, in fact, one of the most infamous psychiatric concentration camps in the United States. Its operation rests on the fact that all its inmates are sentenced to an indeterminate sentence, enhancing the captives' "cooperation" with the captors. The principles animating this institution and the practices carried out in it have received the enthusiastic support of some of the biggest names in American psychiatry—among them, of course, Karl Menninger.[18]

In a class-action suit in 1971, the court, responding to a group of prisoners alleging that they had been subjected to "inhuman treatment," ruled that the use of segregation units at the institution constitutes cruel and unusual punishment. The ruling has led to increased controversy about the methods used at Patuxent. An article in the *APA Monitor* states:

> Psychologist Arthur Kandel, one of Patuxent's three associate directors, testified that the segregation cells (referred to by the inmates as "the hole") were really negative reinforcers . . . used as positive treatment conditions. The court, however, ruled that the physical conditions in the segregation units constituted cruel and unusual punishment. . . . Sigmund Manne, Patuxent's chief psychologist, explains that the indeterminate sentence is "an essential part of the therapeutic program. . . . People respond affectively to the indeterminate sentence," he says. "They don't understand that it's a necessary part of treatment." [19]

In language and law, cure and control are like two banks of a river clearly separated by a body of water—that is, they are clearly separated by a willingness to distinguish between the interests of two parties in conflict with each other. The word *therapy*—as in psychiatric therapy or behavior therapy—is a bridge over the water: it

18. See my *Law, Liberty, and Psychiatry: An Inquiry into the Social Uses of Mental Health Practices* (New York: Macmillan, 1963) and Chapter 9, "Justice in the Therapeutic State," below.

19. S. Trotter, "Patuxent: 'Therapeutic' Prison Faces Test," *APA Monitor* 6 (May 1975): 1.

unites the two parties in a fake cooperation and enables one or the other or both of them to declare the nonexistence of any difference between cure and control, contract and coercion, freedom and slavery.

I have written elsewhere about the debauchment of language in psychiatry and, more particularly, about the use of debauched language by psychiatrists to describe and justify their penological and punitive practices.[20] Psychiatry is now so chock-full of a kind of mental-health newspeak that it is often difficult to know what facts, if any, authors assert. Usually the only thing that is clear is that they insist that what they do is therapeutically effective and morally good. The following quotation from an article entitled "Custody Cases: How Coercive Treatment Works in Kansas City" is typical:

> "Frequently the more disturbed the child, the more severe the psychopathology in the parents and the less able they are to enter voluntarily into a therapeutic alliance," say Paul C. Laybourne, Jr., M.D., director of the [University of Kansas Medical] Center's Division of Child Psychiatry, and associate Janet M. Krueger, A.C.S.W. There may be no such thing as a completely voluntary psychiatric patient under any circumstances, they suggest, supporting their view with a quotation from . . . Richard R. Parlour, M.D.: "Patients are coerced into treatment by pain, fear, and despair as well as by spouses, employers, and judges. Voluntary treatment is a myth."[21]

Here are prominent psychiatrists asserting that two and two makes five and receiving respectable attention for their revelations. Why should that be so? Because they are defending the nobility of the medical faith and the infallibility of the therapeutic papacy, sentiments dear to the hearts of the psychiatric priesthood. But if there is no difference between voluntary and involuntary patienthood, then there is also no difference between voluntary and involuntary servitude. It is only that some people are coerced into working by

20. *Ideology and Insanity: Essays on the Psychiatric Dehumanization of Man* (Garden City, N.Y.: Doubleday, Anchor Press, 1970) and *The Second Sin* (Garden City, N.Y.: Doubleday, Anchor Press, 1973).

21. "Custody Cases: How Coercive Treatment Works in Kansas City," *Roche Report: Frontiers of Hospital Psychiatry*, March 15, 1975, p. 1.

the whip and others by their desire for fame and fortune. That, of course, makes it something of a mystery why slavery should have been opposed and abolished.

The writings of Joseph Wolpe and Arnold Lazarus exhibit a heavy growth of this same semantic fungus. While, on the one hand, they remain discreetly silent about the differences between voluntary and involuntary patients and treatments, on the other, they implicitly endorse the traditional coercions of institutional psychiatry by putting down on paper such sentences as these:

> Some other kinds of corrective statements that commonly need to be made [in behavior therapy] are typified by the following:
>
> 1. You are not mentally ill and there is no chance of your going insane. . . . It is often sufficient to express reassurance in an authoritatively dogmatic way. . . . It must be explained that however bad a neurosis becomes it is still not a psychosis; that psychoses show a clear inherited pattern not manifested in neurosis; that there is evidence of biochemical abnormality in the serum of some psychotics, while neurotics are indistinguishable from normals.[22]

Some people believe that the Jews are the Chosen People; others, that Jesus is the Son of God and is Himself a God; and if Wolpe and Lazarus want to believe what I have quoted in the preceding paragraph, I see no reason to object. After all, it is precisely because they believe and preach those statements that they have been the high priests of behavior therapy.

Wolpe and Lazarus set these "authoritatively dogmatic"—the term is theirs—teachings in their ethical context when they address themselves directly to the moral issues of behavior therapy, where their conclusions are:

> Our discussion of the moral aspects of psychotherapy cannot be concluded without reference to an objection to behavior therapy that is frequently brought up at lectures and seminars, though we do not recall seeing it in print. The complaint is that the behavior therapist assumes a kind of omnipotence in that his methods demand the patient's complete acquiescence, and this, it is felt, denudes the patient of human dignity. The truth is that the grade of acquiescence required

22. J. Wolpe and A. A. Lazarus, *Behavior Therapy Techniques: A Guide to the Treatment of the Neuroses* (New York: Pergamon Press, 1966), p. 19.

> is the same as in any other branch of medicine or education. Patients with pneumonia are ready to do what the medical man prescribes, because he is the expert. The same is the case when psychotherapy is the treatment required.[23]

In short, Wolpe and Lazarus admit—indeed proudly proclaim—that their model for their own therapeutic behavior is the medical man who prescribes treatment for pneumonia.

Leonard Ullmann and Leonard Krasner, both prominent workers in the behavior-therapy movement, have considered specifically the ways in which their views differ from mine. Repeating and remarking on their comments should help to further clarify the issues set before us.

Ullmann briefly summarizes my views on autonomous psychotherapy,[24] cites my statement that "it is the autonomous psychotherapist's responsibility to keep an impenetrable wall between the therapeutic situation and the patient's real life,"and then comments: "The first difference in point of view is that behavior therapy deals with real-life behavior. Work in the home, classroom, ward, and the like facilitates generalization and fosters the changes in behavior which are the target of behavior therapy."[25]

There is a misunderstanding or misrepresentation here between what I mean by "real life" and what Ullmann says I mean by it. I mean quite simply that the therapist must not exert any power outside the consulting room for or against the patient. For example, the therapist may discuss the draft with his patient but may not give him a letter to take to his draft board, or he may discuss suicide with the patient but may not commit him to a hospital to prevent it. In other words, in autonomous psychotherapy the relationship between the therapist and the patient is like that between an architect and the workmen who actually build a house. In each case, the former, no less than the latter, deals with very real things, but he

23. Ibid., p. 23.

24. See my *The Ethics of Psychoanalysis: The Theory and Method of Autonomous Psychotherapy* (New York: Basic Books, 1964).

25. L. P. Ullmann, "Behavior Therapy as Social Movement," in C. M. Franks, ed., *Behavior Therapy: Appraisal and Status* (New York: McGraw-Hill, 1969), p. 513.

deals with them on a verbal or symbolic level—the architect designs a building but does not himself pour concrete. Similarly, the therapist talks about marriage and divorce, conformity and deviance, but does not—and must not—himself make the patient do anything.

In Ullmann's hands my distinctions between the symbolic and the behavioral levels, and between the power of language and law, are transformed into a dichotomy between real and unreal behaviors. Unlike me, behavior therapists, says Ullmann, deal with real-life behavior. By that Ullmann means the actual involvement of behavior therapists in the day-to-day life of the patient. He never uses the word *power*, so it remains unarticulated—though by no means unclear—who will control whom.

The second difference that Ullmann finds between my views and those of behavior therapists is even more astonishing. Let me quote it before commenting on it:

> A second point of difference is the matter of ability to make choices. Because there is only heredity and environment, one must accept the position that any given act, if all antecedents were known, would be determined and completely predictable. . . . In this regard, the individual has no "choice." . . . The concept of choice also poses a logical problem, that of an endless regress. If a person makes a "free choice," what chooses the choice, and what chose that which chooses? Behavior is not completely predictable or determined from the viewpoint of the observer whether that observer is the psychologist or the person himself. The degree of determinism, then, is a function of the theoretical level, and to a lesser extent, of the observer's knowledge. It is paradoxical that the very unpredictability of his behavior may lead the patient to presume that it is determined. . . . There may be real comfort in being powerless and not responsible.[26]

Surely, this is not the place to rehash the controversy over freedom and determinism. I shall therefore try to limit myself to offering a few simple observations.

In the first place, Ullmann is inconsistent even in just this passage (as well as in the whole essay). At the beginning, he asserts that behavior is determined—that people do not make choices. At the end, however, he castigates people who claim that they are

26. Ibid., p. 528.

powerless and not responsible. Although Ullmann qualifies his assertion by saying "in this regard, the individual has no 'choice,' " the individual does have a choice, since "in this regard" refers to conditions that can never be realized. Indeed, Ullmann then explains that "the skill of the therapist is directed toward having the patient make the 'right' choice." Yet only a few pages later he writes: "If the therapist believed in freedom of choice, he could solve this problem. The point of the previous section is that he cannot believe in freedom of choice."[27]

Does Ullmann mean that the therapist *cannot* believe in freedom of choice or that he *must not* believe in it? Obviously, he can believe in it. I do, and I can hardly imagine that I am the only one in the whole world who does. I must confess that I find Ullmann's reasoning and use of language dismaying.

Krasner too considers my position on the ethics of psychotherapeutic influencing, and he, even more sharply than Ullmann, contrasts it with that of the behavior therapists. He joins the issue that I long ago suggested was one of the basic moral premises of psychotherapy—namely, whose agent is the therapist? My view is that the so-called therapist may in fact be the agent of countless individuals and institutions, and that when there are conflicts between them, he must choose whom he proposes to serve. Furthermore, I insist that insofar as the therapist proposes to be a healer, he must be the agent of his patient or client; and that insofar as he proposes to be the agent of society (or of any other individual or group in conflict with the ostensible patient), he ought to recognize, and make explicit, that he functions as the patient's adversary and not as his ally.[28] Here is the way Krasner deals with these issues:

> If it is true that the therapist or modifier of behavior can bring about specified changes in behavior in an individual, on whose behalf is he acting? For whom is the new behavior "good," or desirable, or valuable—for the client, for the therapist, or for society? . . . I could weasel out of this dilemma by some kind of compromise; I could say that I have drawn the issue too sharply, that life is rarely clear-cut,

27. Ibid., pp. 514, 519.
28. See *The Myth of Mental Illness.*

and that the decision is up to the patient. Yet I will not try to avoid this issue and will take a stand that *the therapist is always society's agent.* Szasz takes an apparently opposite point of view in arguing that an individual should have absolute choice over his own behavior, including self-destruction if he so desires. [Italics added[29].]

It would seem from this passage that Krasner is willing to commit the behavior therapist to be an enforcer of social norms and values. However, he declares that that is not what he intends:

> Does this mean that I am developing a picture of a behavior modifier defending the social status quo. . . ? Not at all; in fact, I refer to the view of the therapist himself as an instrument of social change, a modifier of social institutions. In effect the therapist, society's agent, helps change individual behavior and also social institutions themselves.[30]

Sensing the inconsistencies in the views he is propounding, Krasner tries—not very successfully—to resolve them:

> It may look as if behavior modifiers are inconsistent in their view of the relation between society and the individual; in one instance they are agents of society, in the other they denounce society for its rejection of the individual. But these views complement each other. . . . The therapist represents society, but it is a society which is not punitive but rather seeks ways to supply maximum positive social reinforcement to the individual. . . . The good society is one in which all people are positive social reinforcers. The important value is to behave so as to please others and to contribute (as assessed by others) to the general welfare of all men—society. . . . Individuality as unusual, creative, exciting, even unpredictable behaviors elicits positive reinforcement in others, if the behaviors have a social utility, if they are "good" behaviors.[31]

Krasner's whole argument is so weak that I will let most of it speak for itself. His last sentence, however, is so obscenely false that it requires comment. The unusual, creative individual, Krasner declares, "elicits positive reinforcement in others." Socrates and Jesus,

29. L. Krasner, "Behavior Modification—Values and Training: The Perspective of a Psychologist," in Franks, ed., *Behavior Therapy*, pp. 541–542.
30. Ibid., p. 542.
31. Ibid., pp. 543–544.

Spinoza and Semmelweis, would have been interested in this social psychological law. What is one to say when in our day—when perhaps the single most powerful human motive is envy—one of the most prominent American psychologists and behavior therapists asserts that "good" (the quotes are his) behavior elicits positive reinforcement in others? Is this a fatuous tautology or a horrifying assent to Maoism? Either way, I think Krasner here damages the cause of behavior therapy far more than even I would want to.

In the end, it seems to me that behavior therapists cannot easily escape from their own pragmatic strictures, in particular from their own contention that what counts is not what clients or patients say, but what they do: *mutatis mutandis*, what counts is not what behavior modifiers or therapists say, but what they do. Judged by this criterion, behavior therapists are condemned, in my eyes at least, by their uncritical acceptance of the semantic and social consequences of the medicalization of human problems and by their self-serving imposition of behavioral interventions on captive clients. I say this not because I am against behavior therapy, but because I am against therapeutic coercion.

There is, in my mind, an important distinction between not liking something and being opposed to it. I do not like behavior therapy, but I am not opposed to it. I might explain that further by restating what I think behavior modifiers actually do.

Politically speaking, if the behavior therapist has actual—legally legitimized and enforceable—power over the client, then he relieves him of his symptoms in much the same way that the tax collector relieves the citizen of his money. If, on the other hand, he has no such power and his authority over the client derives from the client's own desire for dependency and protection, then the behavior therapist relieves him of his symptoms in much the same way that a church relieves its members of their money.

Psychologically speaking, insofar as in behavior therapy a person is *made* to do something he is afraid to do and hence does not want to do, one of two things must apply—coercion or mock coercion. If the therapist has real power over the patient—for example, if he is a committed mental patient and the therapist has legal authority to "treat" him—then behavior therapy is simply one of the countless ways in which a person who possesses power controls the conduct of another who does not. If, on the other hand, the therapist has no real power over the patient—for example, if the patient is a fee-paying client in a psychologist's private office—then behavior therapy is one of the countless ways in which two persons enact scenes of mock coercion, one of the participants pretending to control, the other pretending to be controlled, and both pretending to believe the other's pretending.

Whether we regard either or both or neither of these uses of behavior therapy as virtuous or wicked will depend, in general, on our ethics and politics and, in particular, on our loyalty, hostility, or indifference to behavior therapy as a psychiatric-psychological method and mystique.

I believe that in the mental-health field, no less than in medicine, our actions should be informed and governed by an ancient Latin maxim and by a fresh amplification of it. The old maxim is *Caveat emptor* ("Let the buyer beware"). The extension of it that I suggest is *Optet emptor* ("Let the buyer choose").

My emphasis is thus on letting the client or patient choose—and benefit or suffer from the consequences of his choice. That is an ethical, not a technical, standard. Hence, my views differ from those of the psychiatric and psychological technicians, whose standard Cole articulates when he declares, "The issue is not whether behavior modification is bad but whether it works."[32] In my view, the issue is not whether behavior modification works but whether the client wants it.

As a rule, a direct confrontation between the technical and the ethical approaches to human affairs is quite unproductive. Each party is interested in something else. The result is an impasse, but perhaps it is an impasse worth restating clearly. The technicist wants to know whether a certain method of intervention in human affairs works or not. It is of course his intervention, and he decides whether it works or not. If it does, he considers it morally good, and it makes no difference what the recipient of his intervention thinks about it.

32. J. O. Cole, "What's in a Word? Or Guilt by Definition, Part I," *Medical Tribune*, June 11, 1975, p. 22.

From that posture, involuntary medical or psychiatric interventions appear good and justifiable, since they are for the benefit of the patient or client. The ethicist wants to know whether a certain method of intervention in human affairs is contracted or coerced. If it is contracted, he concludes that it benefits both parties, although it is likely to be more desirable or necessary for the party that seeks the contract than for the one that accedes to it. If it is coerced, he concludes that it helps the coercer and harms the coerced. From that posture, involuntary medical or psychiatric interventions appear bad and unjustifiable, since they subvert the moral mandate of the helping professions.

Although there may, in actual practice, be a bit more to the moral subtleties of actual psychiatric encounters than is entailed in the foregoing dichotomy, the positions I have pictured point to two important and easily identifiable social roles and personal styles. And the twain shall never meet.

# 6

# The Ethics of Suicide

In 1967, an editorial in the *Journal of the American Medical Association* declared that "the contemporary physician sees suicide as a manifestation of emotional illness. Rarely does he view it in a context other than that of psychiatry."[1] It was implied, the emphasis being the stronger for not being articulated, that to view suicide in this way is at once scientifically accurate and morally uplifting. I shall try to show that it is neither and that, instead, this perspective on suicide is both erroneous and evil—erroneous because it treats an act as if it were a happening and evil because it serves to legitimize psychiatric force and fraud by justifying it as medical care and treatment.

It is difficult to find a "responsible" medical or psychiatric authority today that does not regard suicide as a medical, and specifically as a mental-health, problem.

For example, Ilza Veith, the noted medical historian, declares that "the act [of suicide] clearly represents an illness and is, in fact, the least curable of all diseases." Of course, it was not always thus. Veith herself remarks that "it was only in the nineteenth century that suicide came to be considered a psychiatric illness."[2]

1. Editorial, "Changing Concepts of Suicide," *Journal of the American Medical Association* 199 (March 1967): 162.
2. I. Veith, "Reflections on the Medical History of Suicide," *Modern Medicine*, August 11, 1969, p. 116.

If so, we might ask, What was discovered in the nineteenth century that required removing suicide from the category of sin or crime and putting it into that of illness? The answer is, nothing. Suicide was not *discovered* to be a disease; it was *declared* to be one. The renaming and reclassifying as sick of a whole host of behaviors formerly considered sinful or criminal is the very foundation upon which modern psychiatry rests. I have discussed and documented the process of reclassification elsewhere.[3] Here it should suffice to show how it affects our views on suicide. I shall do so by citing some illustrative opinions.

Bernard R. Shochet, a psychiatrist at the University of Maryland, asserts that "depression is a serious systemic disease, with both physiological and psychological concomitants, and suicide is a part of this syndrome." This claim, as we shall see again and again, serves mainly to justify subjecting the so-called patient to involuntary psychiatric interventions, especially involuntary mental hospitalization: "If the patient's safety is in doubt, psychiatric hospitalization should be insisted on."[4]

Harvey M. Schein and Alan A. Stone, psychiatrists at Harvard University express the same views. "Once the patient's suicidal thoughts are shared," they write, "the therapist must take pains to make clear to the patient that he, the therapist, considers suicide to be a maladaptive action, irreversibly counter to the patient's sane interests and goals; that he, the therapist, will do everything he can to prevent it; and that the potential for such an action arises from the patient's illness. It is equally essential that the therapist believe in the professional stance; if he does not he should not be treating the patient within the delicate human framework of psychotherapy."[5]

It seems to me that if a psychiatrist considers suicide a "maladaptive action," he himself should refrain from engaging in such

3. See my *The Myth of Mental Illness: Foundations of a Theory of Personal Conduct*, rev. ed. (New York: Harper & Row, 1974) and *Ideology and Insanity: Essays on the Psychiatric Dehumanization of Man* (Garden City, N.Y.: Doubleday, Anchor Press, 1970).

4. B. R. Shochet, "Recognizing the Suicidal Patient," *Modern Medicine*, May 18, 1970, pp. 117, 123.

5. H. M. Schein and A. A. Stone, "Psychotherapy Designed to Detect and Treat Suicidal Potential," *American Journal of Psychiatry* 125 (March 1969): 1248–1249.

action. It is not clear why the patient's placing confidence in his therapist to the extent of confiding his suicidal thoughts to him should ipso facto deprive the patient from being the arbiter of his own best interests. Yet this is exactly what Schein and Stone insist on. And again the thrust of the argument is to legitimize depriving the patient of a basic human freedom—the freedom to change therapists when patient and doctor disagree on therapy: "The therapist must insist that patient and physician—*together*—communicate the suicidal potential to important figures in the environment, both professional and family. . . . Suicidal intent must not be part of therapeutic confidentiality." And later, they add: "Obviously this kind of patient must be hospitalized. . . . The therapist must be prepared to step in with hospitalization, with security measures, and with medication. . . .[6] Many other psychiatric authorities could be cited to illustrate the current unanimity on this view of suicide.

Lawyers and jurists have eagerly accepted the psychiatric perspective on suicide, as they have on nearly everything else. An article in the *American Bar Association Journal* by R. E. Schulman, who is both a lawyer and a psychologist, is illustrative. Schulman begins with the premise that no one could claim that suicide is a human right: "No one in contemporary Western society," he writes, "would suggest that people be allowed to commit suicide as they please without some attempt to intervene or prevent such suicides. Even if a person does not value his own life, Western society does value everyone's life."[7]

I should like to suggest, as others have suggested before me, precisely what Schulman claims no one would suggest. Furthermore, if Schulman chooses to believe that Western society—which includes the United States with its history of slavery, Germany with its history of National Socialism, and Russia with its history of Communism—really "does value everyone's life," so be it. But to accept that assertion as true is to fly in the face of the most obvious and brutal facts of history.

Moreover, it is mischievous to put the matter as Schulman phrases it. For it is not necessarily that the would-be suicide "does not value

6. Ibid., pp. 1249, 1250.
7. R. E. Schulman, "Suicide and Suicide Prevention: A Legal Analysis," *American Bar Association Journal* 54 (September 1968): 862.

his own life" but rather that he may no longer want to live it as he must and may value ending it more highly than continuing it.

Schulman, however, has abandoned English for newspeak. That is illustrated by his concluding recommendation regarding treatment. "For those," he writes, "who complete the suicide, that should be the finis as the person clearly intended. For those unsuccessful suicides, the law should uniformly ensure that these people be brought to the attention of the appropriate helping agency. This is not to say that help should be forced upon these people but only that it should be made available. . . ."[8] It is sobering to see such writing in the pages of the *American Bar Association Journal*; it calls to mind what has been dubbed the Eleventh Commandment—"Don't get caught!"

The amazing success of the psychiatric ideology in converting acts into happenings, moral decisions into medical diseases, is thus illustrated by the virtually unanimous acceptance in both medical and legal circles of suicide as an "illness" for which the "patient" is not responsible. If, then, the patient is not responsible for it, someone or something else must be. Psychiatrists and mental hospitals are thus often sued for negligence when a depressed patient commits suicide, and they are often held liable.

How deeply the psychiatric perspective on suicide has penetrated into our culture is shown by the following two cases: in the first, a woman attributed her own suicide attempt to her physician; in the second, a woman attributed her husband's suicide to his employer.

A waitress was given diet pills by a physician to help her lose weight. She then attempted suicide, failed, and sued the physician for giving her a drug that "caused" her to be emotionally upset and attempt suicide. The court held for the physician. But the fact remains that both parties, and the court as well, accepted the underlying thesis—which is what I reject—that attempted suicide is *caused* rather than *willed*. The physician was held not liable, not because the court believed that suicide was a voluntary act, but because the plaintiff failed to show that the defendant was negligent in the "treatment" he prescribed.[9]

8. Ibid.

9. *Fontenot* v. *Tracy*, Super. Ct., San Diego Co., Docket No. 309672 (Cal., 1970); cited in *The Citation* 21 (May 1970): 17–18.

In a similar case, the widow of a ship captain sued the shipping line for the suicide of her husband. She claimed that the captain leaped into the sea because "he was in the grip of an uncontrollable impulse at the time" and that the employer was responsible for that "impulse." Before the case could come to trial, the ship's doctor tried to assert the physician-patient privilege and declined to testify. The court ruled that in a case of this type there was no such privilege under admiralty law. I don't know whether or not the plaintiff has ultimately succeeded in her suit. But again, whatever the outcome, the proposition that suicide is an event brought about by certain antecedent *causes* rather than that it is an act motivated by certain *desires* (in this case, perhaps the ship captain's wish not to be reunited with his wife) is here enshrined in the economics, law, and semantics of a civil suit for damages.[10]

When a person decides to take his life and when a physician decides to frustrate him in this action, the question arises, Why should the physician do so?

Conventional psychiatric wisdom answers, Because the suicidal person suffers from a mental illness whose symptom is his desire to kill himself; it is the physician's duty to diagnose and treat illness; ergo, he must prevent the patient from killing himself and at the same time must treat the underlying disease that causes the patient to wish to do away with himself. That looks like an ordinary medical diagnosis and intervention. But it is not. What is missing? Everything. The hypothetical suicidal patient is not ill: he has no demonstrable bodily disorder (or if he does, it does not cause his suicide); he does not assume the sick role—he does not seek medical help. In short, the physician uses the rhetoric of illness and treatment to justify his forcible intervention in the life of a fellow human being—often in the face of explicit opposition from his so-called patient.

I object to that as I do to all involuntary psychiatric interventions, and especially involuntary mental hospitalization. I have de-

10. *Reid* v. *Moore-McCormack Lines, Inc.*, Dist. Ct., N.Y., Docket No. 69 Civ. 1259 (D.C., N.Y., January 15, 1970); cited in *The Citation* 21 (May 1970): 31.

tailed my reasons why elsewhere and need not repeat them here.[11] For the sake of emphasis, however, let me state that I consider counseling, persuasion, psychotherapy, or any other voluntary measure, especially for persons troubled by their own suicidal inclinations and seeking such help, unobjectionable, and indeed generally desirable. However, physicians and psychiatrists are usually not satisfied with limiting their help to such measures—and with good reason: from such assistance the individual may gain not only the desire to live, but also the strength to die.

However, we still have not answered the question posed above, Why should a physician frustrate an individual from killing himself? Some might answer, Because the physician values the patient's life, at least when the patient is suicidal, more highly than does the patient himself. Let us examine that claim. Why should the physician, often a complete stranger to the suicidal patient, value the patient's life more highly than does the patient himself? He does not do so in medical practice. Why then should he do so in psychiatric practice, which he himself insists is a form of medical practice? Let us assume that a physician is confronted with an individual suffering from diabetes or heart failure who fails to take the drugs prescribed for his illness. We know that that can happen, and we know what happens in such cases—the patient does not do as well as he might, and he may die prematurely. Yet it would be absurd for a physician to consider, much less to attempt, taking over the conduct of such a patient's life, confining him in a hospital against his will in order to treat his disease. Indeed, an attempt to do so would bring the physician into conflict with both the civil and the criminal law. For, significantly, the law recognizes the medical patient's autonomy despite the fact that, unlike the suicidal individual, he suffers from a real disease and despite the fact that, unlike the nonexistent disease of the suicidal individual, his illness is often easily controlled by simple and safe therapeutic procedures.

Nevertheless, the threat of alleged or real suicide, or so-called dangerousness to oneself, is everywhere considered a proper ground

11. See my *Law, Liberty, and Psychiatry: An Inquiry into the Social Uses of Mental Health Practices* (New York: Macmillan, 1963) and *Ideology and Insanity*, esp. chaps. 9 and 12.

and justification for involuntary mental hospitalization and treatment. Why should that be so?

Surely, the answer cannot be that the physician values the suicidal individual's life more highly than does that individual himself. If he really did, he could prove it—and indeed would have to prove it—by the means we usually employ to judge such matters. Here are some examples.

Because of famine, a family is starving: the parents go without food and may perish so that their children might survive. A boat is shipwrecked and is sinking: the captain goes down with the ship so that his passengers might survive.

Were the physician sincere in his claim that he values the would-be suicide's life so highly, should we not expect him to prove it by some similar act of self-sacrifice? A person may be suicidal because he has lost his money. Does the psychiatrist give him his money? Certainly not. Another may be suicidal because he is alone in the world. Does the psychiatrist give him his friendship? Certainly not.

Actually, the suicide-preventing psychiatrist does not give anything of his own to his patient. Instead, he uses the claim that he values the suicidal individual's life more highly than that individual does himself to justify his self-serving strategies; the psychiatrist aggrandizes himself as a *suicidologist*—as if new words were enough to create new wisdoms—and he enlists the economic and police powers of the state on his own behalf, using tax monies to line his own pockets and to hire underlings to take care of his patient, and psychiatric violence to guarantee himself a patient upon whom to work his medical miracles.

Let me suggest what I believe is likely to be the most important reasón for the profound antisuicidal bias of the medical profession. Physicians are committed to saving lives. How then should they react to people who are committed to throwing away their lives? It is natural for people to dislike, indeed to hate, those who challenge their basic values. The physician thus reacts, perhaps "unconsciously" (in the sense that he does not articulate the problem in these terms) to the suicidal patient as if the patient had affronted, insulted, or attacked him. The physician strives valiantly, often at the cost of his own well-being, to save lives; and here comes a person who not only does not let the physician save him but, *horribile dictu*, makes the physician an unwilling witness to that person's deliberate self-destruction. That is more than most physicians can take. Feeling assaulted in the very center of their spiritual identity, some take to flight, while others counterattack.

Some physicians will thus avoid dealing with suicidal patients. That explains why many people who end up killing themselves have a record of having consulted a physician, often on the very day of their suicide. I surmise that those people go in search of help only to discover that the physician wants nothing to do with them. And in a sense it is right that it should be so. I do not blame the doctors. Nor do I advocate teaching them suicide prevention—whatever that might be. I contend that because physicians have a relatively blind faith in their lifesaving ideology—which, moreover, they often need to carry them through their daily work—they are the wrong people for listening and talking to individuals intelligently and calmly about suicide. So much for those physicians who, in the face of the existential attack that they feel the suicidal patient launches on them, run for their lives. Let us now look at those who stand and fight back.

Some physicians (and other mental-health professionals) declare themselves ready and willing to help not only suicidal patients who seek assistance, but all persons who are, or are alleged to be, suicidal. Since they too seem to perceive suicide as a threat, not just to the suicidal person's physical survival but to their own value system, they strike back and strike back hard. That explains why psychiatrists and suicidologists resort, apparently with a perfectly clear conscience, to the vilest means: they must believe that their lofty ends justify the basest means. Hence, we have the prevalent use of force and fraud in suicide prevention. The upshot of that kind of interaction between physician and patient is a struggle for power. The patient is at least honest about what he wants: to gain control over his life and death—by being the agent of his own demise. But the psychiatrist is completely dishonest about what he wants: he claims that he only wants to help his patient, but actually he wants to gain control over the patient's life in order to save himself from having to confront his doubts about the value of his own life. Suicide is medical heresy. Commitment and electroshock are the appropriate psychiatric-inquisitorial remedies for it.

Like politicians, psychiatrists must often choose between being popular and being honest; though they may strive valiantly to be both, they are not likely to succeed. There are good reasons why that should be so. Men need rules to live by. They need authority they can respect and that is capable of compelling conformity to rules. Hence, institutions, even institutions ostensibly devoted to the study of human affairs, are much better at articulating rules than at analyzing them. I shall illustrate the relevance of these remarks to our attitude toward suicide by citing the recent history of our attitudes toward contraception and abortion. For birth control and abortion, like suicide, are matters that touch on religion and law as well as on medicine and psychiatry.

Although it was widely practiced, birth control was regarded as vaguely reprehensible until well past the Second World War. Only in 1965 did the Supreme Court strike down as unconstitutional a Connecticut statute against the dissemination of birth-control information and devices.[12]

In 1959, I polled the opinion of members of the American Psychoanalytic Association on several topics, some pertaining to the moral aspects of psychoanalytic practices. Among the questions I asked was, "Do you believe that birth-control information should be unrestrictedly available to all persons eighteen years of age and over?" The questionnaire, which was to be returned unsigned, was sent to 752 psychoanalysts; 430, or 56 percent, replied. Thirty-four analysts, or 9 percent of those responding, asserted that they did *not* believe that adult Americans should have free access to birth-control information.[13]

In this connection, it is significant that only in 1964 did the House of Delegates of the American Medical Association approve a resolution endorsing the general availability of contraceptive information and measures. Until that time, the American Medical Association *opposed* free access by American adults to birth control information!

The story about abortion is similar. In my poll, I also asked, "Do you regard the legally restricted availability of abortion as socially

12. *Griswold* v. *Connecticut*, 381 U.S. 479 (1965).

13. T. S. Szasz and R. A. Nemiroff, "A Questionnaire Study of Psychoanalytic Practices and Opinions," *Journal of Nervous and Mental Diseases* 137 (September 1963): 209–221.

desirable?" Two hundred and two, or nearly 50 percent of the analysts who responded, opposed the repeal of legal restrictions on abortion. (Only seven analysts identified themselves as Roman Catholics.)[14]

In 1965, the year after the Committee on Human Reproduction of the American Medical Association recommended the resolution on contraception just mentioned, it introduced a proposal for more "liberal" abortion laws—that is, for laws expanding the medical and psychiatric grounds for therapeutic abortions. The House of Delegates refused to approve that recommendation. Without discussion or dissent, the delegates agreed that "it is not appropriate at this time for the American Medical Association to recommend the enactment of legislation in this matter."[15]

In 1970, after New York State removed abortion from the purview of the criminal law, the American Psychoanalytic Association issued its "Position Statement on Abortion" affirming that "We view a therapeutic abortion as a medical procedure to be agreed upon between a patient and her physician; and one which should be removed entirely from the domain of the criminal law."[16]

The point I am making here, and have been making for some time, is simply that contraception and abortion, and suicide too, are not medical but moral problems. To be sure, the procedure of aborting a pregnancy is surgical; but that makes abortion no more a medical problem than the use of the electric chair makes capital punishment a problem of electrical engineering. The question is, What is abortion—the killing of a fetus or the removal of a piece of tissue from a woman's body?

Likewise, it is undeniable that suicide, if successful, results in death. But if the suicidal act is regarded as a disease because it is the proximate cause of death, then all other acts or events—from highway traffic to avalanches, from poverty to war—that may also be the proximate causes of death would also have to be regarded as diseases. Just so, say the modern manufacturers of madness, the

14. Ibid., p. 214.

15. Quoted in my "The Ethics of Abortion," *The Humanist* 26 (September–October): 147.

16. American Psychoanalytic Association, "Position Statement on Abortion," May 7, 1970.

community psychiatrists and the epidemiologists of mental illness, who push tirelessly for a 100 percent incidence of mental illness.[17] I say all that is malicious nonsense.

In the non-Communist West, opposition to suicide, like opposition to contraception and abortion, rests on religious grounds. According to both the Jewish and Christian religions, God created man, and man can use himself only in the ways permitted by God. Preventing conception, aborting a pregnancy, or killing oneself are, in this imagery, all sins: each is a violation of the laws laid down by God or by theological authorities claiming to speak in his name.

But modern man is a revolutionary. Like all revolutionaries, he likes to take away from those who have and to give to those who have not, especially himself. He has thus taken man from God and given him to the state (with which he often identifies more than he knows). That is why the state gives and takes away so many of our rights and why we consider the arrangement whereby the state stands *in loco parentis* to the citizen-child so natural. (Hence, the linguistic abomination of referring to the abolition of prohibittions, say, against abortion or off-track betting, as the *legalizing* of these acts.)

But this arrangement leaves suicide in a peculiar moral and philosophical limbo. For if a man's life belongs to the state (as it formerly belonged to God), then surely suicide is the taking of a life that belongs not to the taker but to the state.

The dilemma this simplistic transfer of body ownership from God to state raises derives from the fundamental difference between a religious and a secular world view, especially when the former entails a vivid conception of a life after death and the latter does not (or even emphatically repudiates it). More particularly, the dilemma derives from the problem of how to punish successful suicide. Traditionally, the Roman Catholic Church punished it by depriving the suicide of burial in consecrated ground. As far as I know, that practice is now so rare in the United States as to be prac-

17. See my *The Myth of Mental Illness*, esp. pp. 38–39.

tically nonexistent. Suicides are now given a Catholic burial, as they are routinely considered to have taken their lives while insane.

The modern state, with psychiatry as its secular-religious ally, has no comparable sanction to offer. Could that be one of the reasons why it punishes so severely—so very much more severely than did the church—the unsuccessful suicide? For I consider the psychiatric stigmatization of people as "suicidal risks" and their incarceration in psychiatric institutions a form of punishment, and a very severe one at that. Indeed, although I cannot support the claim with statistics, I believe that accepted psychiatric methods of suicide prevention often aggravate rather than ameliorate the suicidal person's problems. As one reads of the tragic encounters with psychiatry of such people as James Forrestal, Marilyn Monroe, or Ernest Hemingway, one gains the impression that they felt demeaned and deeply hurt by the psychiatric indignities inflicted on them and that as a result of those experiences they were even more desperately driven to suicide. In short, I am suggesting that coerced psychiatric interventions may increase, rather than diminish, the suicidal person's desire for self-destruction.

But there is another aspect of the moral and philosophical dimensions of suicide that must be mentioned here. I refer to the growing influence of the modern idea of individualism, especially the conviction that human beings have certain inalienable rights. Some people have thus come to believe (or perhaps only to believe that they believe) that they have a right to life, liberty, and property. That makes for some interesting complications for the modern legal and psychiatric stand on suicide.

The individualistic position on suicide might be put thus: A person's life belongs to himself. Hence, he has a right to take his own life, that is, to commit suicide. To be sure, this view recognizes that a person may also have a moral responsibility to his family and others and that, by killing himself, he reneges on these responsibilities. But those are moral wrongs that society, in its corporate capacity as the state, cannot properly punish. Hence, the state must eschew attempts to regulate such behavior by means of formal sanctions, such as criminal or mental-hygiene laws.

The analogy between life and property lends further support to this line of argument. Having a right to property means that a person can dispose of it even if in so doing he injures himself and his family. A man may give, or gamble, away his money. But, significantly, he cannot be said to steal from himself. The concept of theft requires at least two parties—one who steals and another from whom something is stolen. There is no such thing as *self-theft*. The term *suicide* blurs that very distinction. The history of the term indicates that suicide was long considered a type of homicide. Indeed, when a person wants to condemn suicide, he calls it *self-murder*. Schulman, for example, writes, "Surely, self-murder falls within the province of the law."[18]

Some of the results of my poll are of interest in this connection. In it, I asked two questions about suicide. One was, "In your opinion, how often is a *successful* suicide (in contemporary Western democracies) a rational act motivated by the wish to die?" The other was the same question about *unsuccessful* suicide. Of the 430 analysts responding, only 2, or 0.5 percent, thought that successful suicide was always a rational act, and only a single analyst, or 0.25 percent, thought that unsuccessful suicide was. There were only 2 more respondents who thought that successful suicide was a rational act in over 75 percent of the cases and 2 who thought that unsuccessful suicide was a rational act in over 75 percent of the cases. The overwhelming number of respondents, approximately 80 percent for both questions, expressed the view that both successful and unsuccessful suicide is either never a rational act or is such in less than 5 percent of all cases.[19] In short, psychoanalysts came down squarely for viewing suicidal behavior, attempted or completed, as something irrational—that is, a symptom of mental illness. It is upon such confused and confusing images of suicide that our contemporary psychiatric practices of suicide prevention are based.

The suicidologist has a literally schizophrenic view of the suicidal person: he sees him as two persons in one, each at war with the other. One half of the patient wants to die; the other half wants to live. The former, says the suicidologist, is wrong; the latter is right. And he proceeds to protect the latter by restraining the former. How-

18. Schulman, "Suicide and Suicide Prevention," p. 857.
19. Szasz and Nemiroff, "Questionnaire," p. 214.

ever, since these two people are, like Siamese twins, one, he can restrain the suicidal half only by restraining the whole person.

The absurdity of the medical-psychiatric position on suicide does not end here. It ends in extolling mental health and physical survival over every other value, particularly individual liberty. In regarding the desire to live, but not the desire to die, as a legitimate human aspiration, the suicidologist stands Patrick Henry's famous exclamation, "Give me liberty, or give me death!" on its head. In effect, he says, "*Give him* commitment, *give him* electroshock, *give him* lobotomy, *give him* lifelong slavery, but *do not let him choose* death!" By so radically illegitimizing another person's (but not his own) wish to die, the suicide-preventer redefines the aspiration of the Other as not an aspiration at all: the wish to die becomes something an irrational, mentally diseased being *displays* or something that *happens* to a lower form of life. The result is a far-reaching infantilization and dehumanization of the suicidal person.

For example, Phillip Solomon writes that physicians "must protect the patient from his own [suicidal] wishes"; while to Edwin Schneidman, "Suicide prevention is like fire prevention."[20] Solomon thus reduces the would-be suicide to the level of an unruly child, while Schneidman reduces him to the level of a tree! In short, the suicidologist uses his professional stance to illegitimize and punish the wish to die.

There is of course nothing new about any of this. Do-gooders have always opposed personal autonomy or self-determination. In "Amok," written in 1931, Stefan Zweig puts these words into the mouth of his protagonist:

> Ah, yes, "It's one's duty to help." That's your favorite maxim, isn't it? . . . Thank you for your good intentions, but I'd rather be left to myself. . . . So I won't trouble you to call, if you don't mind. Among the "rights of man" there is a right which no one can take away, the right to croak when and where and how one pleases, without a "helping hand."[21]

20. P. Solomon, "The Burden of Responsibility in Suicide," *Journal of the American Medical Association* 199 (January 1967): 324; E. Schneidman, "Preventing Suicide," *Bulletin of Suicidology* (1968): 20.

21. S. Zweig, "Amok," in his *The Royal Game* (New York: Viking, 1944), p. 137.

But that is not the way the scientific psychiatrist or suicidologist sees the problem. He might agree (I suppose) that in the abstract man has the right Zweig claimed for him. But in practice suicide (so he says) is the result of insanity, madness, mental illness. Furthermore, it makes no sense to say that one has a right to be mentally ill, especially if the illness is one that, like typhoid fever, threatens the health of other people as well. In short, the suicidologist's job is to try to convince people that wanting to die is a disease.

Here is how Ari Kiev, director of the Cornell Program in Social Psychiatry and its suicide prevention clinic, does it:

> We say [to the patient], look, you have a disease, just like the Hong Kong flu. Maybe you've got the Hong Kong depression. First, you've got to realize you are emotionally ill. . . . Most of the patients have never admitted to themselves that they are sick.[22]

This pseudomedical perspective is then used to justify psychiatric deceptions and coercions of the crudest sort. For example, here is the way, according to the *Wall Street Journal*, the Los Angeles Suicide Prevention Center operates. A man calls and says he is about to shoot himself. The worker asks for his address. The man refuses to give it.

> "If I pull it [the trigger] now I'll be dead," he [the caller] said in a muffled voice. "And that's what I want." Silently but urgently, Mrs. Whitbook [the worker] had signalled a co-worker to begin tracing the call. And now she worked to keep the man talking. . . . An agonizing 40 minutes passed. Then she heard the voice of a policeman come on the phone to say the man was safe.[23]

But surely, if this man was able to call the Suicide Prevention Center, he could have, had he wanted to, called for a policeman himself; but he did not. He was deceived by the center in the "service" he got. Evidently, those who practice in this way—and such medical deception is of course time honored—believe that the ends, at least in their case, justify the means.

I understand that this kind of deception is standard practice in suicide prevention centers, though it is often denied that it is. A

22. *The New York Times*, February 9, 1969.
23. *The Wall Street Journal*, March 6, 1969.

report about the Nassau County Suicide Prevention Service corroborates the impression that when the would-be suicide does not cooperate with the suicide-prevention authorities, he is confined involuntarily. "When a caller is obviously suicidal," we are told, "a Meadowbrook ambulance is sent out immediately to pick him up."[24]

One more example of the sort of thing that goes on in the name of suicide prevention should suffice. It is a routine story from a Syracuse newspaper about a potential suicide. The gist of it is all in one sentence: "A 28-year-old Minoa [a Syracuse suburb] man was arrested last night on a charge of violation of the Mental Health Law after police authorities said they spent two hours looking for him in a Minoa woods."[25] But why should the police look for such a man? Why not wait until he returns? Those are rhetorical questions. Our answers to them depend on, and reflect, our concepts of what it means to be a human being: That is the crux of the matter.

The crucial contradiction about suicide viewed as an illness whose treatment is a medical responsibility is that suicide is an action but is treated as if it were a happening. As I showed elsewhere, that contradiction lies at the heart of all so-called mental illnesses or psychiatric problems.[26] However, it poses a particularly acute dilemma for suicide, because suicide is the only fatal "mental illness."

Before concluding, I should like to restate briefly my views on the differences between diseases and desires and show that, by persisting in treating desires as diseases, we only end up treating man as a slave.

Let us take as our paradigm case of illness a skier who takes a bad spill and fractures an ankle. The fracture is something that has happened to him; he has not intended it to happen. (To be sure, he may have intended it, but that is another case.) Once it has happened, he will seek medical help and will cooperate with medical efforts to mend his broken bones. In short, the person and his fractured ankle are, as it were, two separate entities, the former acting on the latter.

24. See "Clinic Moves to Prevent Suicides in Suburbia," *Medical World News*, July 28, 1967, p. 17.

25. *Syracuse Post-Standard*, September 29, 1969.

26. *The Myth of Mental Illness.*

Let us now consider the case of the suicidal person. Such a person may also look upon his own suicidal inclination as an undesired, almost alien, impulse and seek help to combat it. If so, the ensuing arrangement between him and his psychiatrist is readily assimilated to the standard medical model of treatment: the patient actively seeks and cooperates with professional efforts to remedy his "condition." As I already noted, I have neither moral nor psychiatric objection to that arrangement. On the contrary, I wholly approve of it.

But as we have seen, that is not the only way, nor perhaps the most important way, that the game of suicide prevention is played. It is accepted medical and psychiatric practice to treat people for their suicidal desires against their will. And what exactly does that mean? It means something quite different from the involuntary (or nonvoluntary) treatment of a bodily illness that is often given as an analogy. For a fractured ankle can be set whether or not a patient consents to its being set. It can be done because setting a fracture is a *mechanical act on the body*. But preventing suicide—suicide being the result of human desire and action—requires a *political act on the person*. In other words, since suicide is an exercise and expression of human freedom, it can be prevented only by curtailing human freedom. That is why deprivation of liberty becomes, in institutional psychiatry, a form of treatment.

In the final analysis, the would-be suicide is like the would-be emigrant: both want to leave where they are and move elsewhere. The suicide wants to leave life and move on to death. The emigrant wants to leave his homeland and move on to another country.

Let us take the analogy seriously; after all, it is much more faithful to the facts than is the analogy between suicide and illness. A crucial characteristic that distinguishes open from closed societies is that people are free to leave the former but not the latter. The medical profession's stance on suicide is thus like the Communists' on emigration: the doctors insist that the would-be suicide survive, just as the Russians insist that the would-be emigrant stay home.

The true believer in Communism is convinced that in the Soviet Union everything belongs to the people and everything done is done for their benefit: anyone who would want to leave such a country must be mad—or bad. In either case, he must be prevented from doing so. Similarly, the true believer in Medicine is convinced that, with modern science guarding their well-being, people have opportunities for a happy and healthy life such as they never had before: anyone who would want to leave such a life prematurely must be mad—or bad. In either case, he must be prevented from doing so.

In short, I submit that preventing people from killing themselves is like preventing people from leaving their homeland. Whether those who so curtail other people's liberties act with complete sincerity or with utter cynicism hardly matters. What matters is what happens—the abridgement of individual liberty, justified, in the case of suicide prevention, by psychiatric rhetoric; and, in the case of emigration prevention, by political rhetoric.

In language and logic, we are the prisoners of our premises, just as in politics and law we are the prisoners of our rulers. Hence, we had better pick them well. For if suicide is an illness because it terminates in death, and if the prevention of death by any means necessary is the physician's therapeutic mandate, then the proper remedy for suicide is indeed liberticide.

# 7

# Language and Lunacy

I must confess that I am not sure any more what the term *humanism* means. I know, of course, that all of us here are humanists and that it is good to be a humanist. But frankly I am troubled by that sort of use of the term *humanism*—that is, by the fact that humanism implies an idea or ideal that no one—in his right mind, if I may put it that way—can be against. I think we should try to transcend humanism as a mere rhetoric of self-approbation and give it a stricter meaning.

Although you may accept the necessity of this task without further discussion, let me cite in support of my foregoing assertion the principal definitions of humanism offered by *Webster's Third New International Dictionary*: ". . . (2) devotion to human welfare: interest in or concern for man (3) a doctrine, set of attitudes, or way of life centered upon human interests and values: as (*a*) a philosophy that rejects supernaturalism, regards man as a natural object, and asserts the essential dignity and worth of man and his capacity to achieve self-realization through the use of reason and scientific method—called also *naturalistic humanism, scientific humanism* . . . (*c*) a philosophy advocating the self-fulfillment of man within the framework of Christian principles—called also *Christian humanism. . . .*"

The first three characterizations of humanism are so framed as to command nearly universal assent; why should anyone be opposed to a "concern for man"? The fourth definition narrows the field to those who reject fundamentalistic religions; and the fifth, to those who embrace Christianity. None of them are of much help. Moreover, there are those who speak of *socialist humanism, existentialist humanism*, and so forth—each of those terms referring to views of the world, and of man in it, from the particular normative perspective of the speaker and his ethical system. The term *humanism* in most of those contexts and phrases is simply a tautology. That contention is supported by the fact that no one, to my knowledge, has ever advocated an ethic of inhumanism or has ever called himself an *inhumanist.*

All this points to the importance of language in coming to grips with what is humanism, or at least with what we want to say about it in such a way as to render both assent to it and dissent from it intelligible and, at least in principle, respectable.

Although the contemporary concept of humanism is shrouded in considerable confusion and controversy, the humanists of the past—particularly those of Athens and Rome, and of the Renaissance and the Enlightenment—are like stars in the firmament with whose aid we can steer our course through the troubled seas of modern ideologies. Moreover, although books—and, indeed, whole lives—have been devoted to the exploration and exposition of those bygone humanisms and humanists, it is fair to say that those great epochs and their representative thinkers shared one characteristic—namely, an abiding concern for language and, more specifically, a concern for individual freedom as expressed by clear and forthright speech and for self-restraint as expressed by the disciplined and aesthetic use of language. A few illustrations, to convey the spirit rather than the substance of this outlook on life, will have to suffice here.

"A slave," said Euripides, "is he who cannot speak his thought." The right of a citizen to say what he pleased was fundamental in Athens. The Greeks, Edith Hamilton tells us, "had no authoritative Sacred Book, no creed, no ten commandments, no dogmas. The very idea of orthodoxy was unknown to them."[1] This pervasive sense of

1. E. Hamilton, *The Greek Way to Western Civilization* (New York: New American Library, Mentor, 1958), p. 208.

spiritual freedom and responsibility enabled the Greeks to see the world clearly: hence their unsurpassed power as artists, whether in fashioning stones or words. In Rome, Cicero, Seneca, and Plutarch continued the Greek tradition of humanism, laying the foundations for the ground on which, fifteen centuries later, the Enlightenment humanists made their stand and from which they drew their initial sustenance. *"Homo res sacra homini"* ("Man is a sacred thing to man"), said Seneca, who, in his own life, labored to oppose the fraudulent rhetoric of demagogy with clear and simple speech.

The modern age and, with it, modern humanism were ushered in with the rediscovery of the ancient classics, with the struggles that accompanied the translations of the Bible into the "vulgar" European tongues, and with the reemphasis by the *philosophes* of the intimate connection between clear thought and clear speech.

Both classical and Renaissance humanists thus displayed deep concern not only for human freedom and dignity but also for the disciplined and honest use of language. The essential, perhaps even organic, unity between man and his language has been severed in the modern age, with many contemporary humanists displaying unconcern for language and many contemporary students of language displaying unconcern for humanism.

In proportion, then, as a person uses language poorly or well, he thinks poorly or well; and, accordingly, we tend to attribute a diminished or enhanced human stature to him. Children, uneducated people, foreigners, and madmen thus tend to be seen as possessing a diminished human stature; whereas novelists, playwrights, composers, philosophers, and scientists tend to be seen as possessing an enhanced human stature. I am not asserting that the proper or accomplished use of language is sufficient for qualifying a person as a humanist, but I am suggesting that it may be necessary for it.

In short, I believe there is a pressing need among contemporary humanists for a fresh emphasis on language; for although rationality, reasoning, and thinking occupy important positions in the modern humanist credo, language, writing, and speaking are conspicuous by their absence from it. But it is idle, or worse, to persist in characterizing people according to how they reason when all that we can observe is how they use language.

To illustrate and support my suggestion that there is a grave danger in connecting humanism with reason rather than with language, I have chosen the example of Eugen Bleuler's perception of certain of the inhabitants of insane asylums, whom he called *schizophrenics*. That perception is, as I shall try to show, gravely mistaken.

It might be best, before turning to Bleuler's views on schizophrenia, to state briefly the current, generally accepted definition. Schizophrenia is said to be a "mental disease whose principal manifestation or symptom is a disturbance of thinking."[2] And what is thinking? Here is how the author of one of the standard American textbooks of psychiatry defines it: "The joining of ideas one to another by imagining, conceiving, inferring, and other processes, and the formation of new ideas by these processes, constitute the function we know as thinking. . . . Thought is the most highly organized of psychobiological integrations."[3]

That sort of pretentious psychiatric jargon seeks to conceal the observable facts of speech behind the abstract concept of thought. Modern psychiatry has accepted the notion of thought as if it were like liver or kidney and has erected a complex system of psychopathology upon it. In that way, psychiatrists have generated a whole catalogue of "disorders of thinking," among which they list such things as incoherence, delusions, hypochondria, obsessions, and phobias. But the communications to which these terms refer (if they refer to anything at all and are not used simply to stigmatize people whose language-behavior does not differ noticeably from that of others) are disorders only in the sense that they offend the patient's relatives, "normal" people, or psychiatrists. My point—a point that has been made by others, especially since Freud and Jung—is that so-called mental patients do not talk gibberish. To be sure, sometimes they talk differently than others do. Sometimes they say things that offend others. In short, they speak—just as do you and I—though perhaps in accents and metaphors that we do not understand or, if we understand them, that we do not like.

2. American Psychiatric Association, *Diagnostic and Statistical Manual of Mental Disorders*, 2d ed. (Washington, D.C.: American Psychiatric Association, 1968), p. 33.

3. L. C. Kolb, *Noyes' Modern Clinical Psychiatry*, 7th ed. (Philadelphia: Saunders, 1968), p. 95.

I have tried to suggest some connections among the notions of thinking, reasoning, speaking, language, and being human. Since I am a psychiatrist (of sorts); since so-called schizophrenic persons have, because of the disease from which they allegedly suffer, been regarded as not fully human; and since that disease is said to be a disorder, above all else, of thinking, I think you will agree that it is appropriate if I attend more closely to that mysterious disease. However, since I consider the disease to be mythical or nonexistent, I cannot attend to it as if it existed in nature; [4] instead, I will consider the account given of it by its inventor, Eugen Bleuler.

In 1911, Bleuler published the monograph *Dementia Praecox, or the Group of Schizophrenias*, which made him famous. In it, he proposes the name *schizophrenia* for a "group of diseases" characterized by certain patterns of behavior and speech on the part of the patient whom Bleuler considered pathological. "I call dementia praecox 'schizophrenia,' " he wrote, "because . . . the 'splitting' of the different psychic functions is one of its most important characteristics."[5] Since no one has seen or will ever see a psychic function, split or unsplit, Bleuler here speaks metaphorically. Yet, as I shall show in a moment, when the alleged patient speaks metaphorically, Bleuler calls him schizophrenic.

But here, first, is Bleuler's own definition of schizophrenia:

> By the term "dementia praecox" or "schizophrenia" we designate a group of psychoses whose course is at times chronic, at times marked by intermittent attacks, and which can stop or retrograde at any state, but does not permit a full *restitutio ad integrum*. The disease is characterized by a specific type of alteration of thinking.[6]

That is how, in 1911, the earlier notion that lunatics are irrational is rehabilitated and given fresh scientific legitimacy: madness becomes schizophrenia, a disease characterized by disordered thinking.

One does not need to know any psychiatry but only to have some

4. See my "The Problem of Psychiatric Nosology," *American Journal of Psychiatry* 114 (November 1957): 405–413, and *Schizophrenia: The Sacred Symbol of Psychiatry* (New York: Basic Books, 1976).

5. E. Bleuler, *Dementia Praecox, or the Group of Schizophrenias*, trans. Joseph Zinkin (New York: International Uuniversities Press, 1950), p. 8.

6. Ibid., p. 9.

respect for the proper use of language to appreciate that the psychiatrist's *thinking* is like the physicist's *ether*; it is an abstraction created to talk about observable things, such as speaking and writing. Indeed Bleuler's book is full of illustrations of the utterances, pleas, letters, and other linguistic productions of so-called schizophrenic patients. And he himself offers numerous remarks about language, such as the following: "Blocking, poverty of ideas, incoherence, clouding, delusions, and emotional anomalies are expressed in the language of the patients. However, the abnormality does not lie in the language itself, but rather in its content." [7]

Bleuler goes to great effort to protect himself against creating the impression that in describing a schizophrenic patient he is merely describing someone who speaks oddly, or differently than he does, and with whom he, Bleuler, disagrees. He never ceases to emphasize that such is not the case—that the patient is sick and his linguistic behavior is only a symptom of his illness. Here is one of Bleuler's statements epitomizing this line of argument:

> The form of linguistic expression may show every imaginable abnormality, or be absolutely correct. We often find very convincing ways of speaking in intelligent individuals. At times, I was unable to convince all of my audience attending clinical demonstrations of the pathology of such severely schizophrenic logic.[8]

Bleuler's premise here precludes—and seems intended to preclude—questioning *whether* the person in question is sick. We are allowed to question only *how* he is sick—what sort of illness he has, what sort of pathology his thinking exhibits. To assent to that is, of course, to give away the game before beginning to play it.

Frequently, the only thing wrong (as it were) with the so-called schizophrenic is that he speaks in metaphors unacceptable to his audience, in particular to his psychiatrist. Sometimes Bleuler comes close to acknowledging that. For example, he writes that

> a patient says that he is being "subjected to rape," although his confinement in a mental hospital constitutes a different kind of violation of his person. To a large extent, *inappropriate figures of speech* are

7. Ibid., p. 147.
8. Ibid., p. 148.

> employed, particularly the word "murder" which recurs constantly for all forms of torment and in the most varied combinations. [Italics added.] [9]

Here we have a rare opportunity to see how language displays what is quintessentially human and at the same time to see how language may be used to deprive individuals of their humanity. When persons imprisoned in mental hospitals speak of *rape* and *murder*, they use inappropriate figures of speech that signify that they suffer from thought disorders; when psychiatrists call their prisons *hospitals*, their prisoners *patients*, and their patients' desire for liberty *disease*, the psychiatrists are not using figures of speech but are stating facts.

The remarkable thing about all of this is that Bleuler understood perfectly well, probably much better than do many psychiatrists today, that much of what appears strange or objectionable in schizophrenic language is the way such persons use metaphor. Nevertheless, he felt justified, on the ground of that fact and that alone, in regarding such persons as suffering from a disease—in the literal rather than metaphorical sense. "When one patient declares," writes Bleuler,

> that she is Switzerland, or when another wants to take a bunch of flowers to bed with her so that she will not awaken any more—these utterances seem to be quite incomprehensible at first glance. But we obtain a key to the explanation by virtue of the knowledge that these patients readily substitute similarities for identities and think in symbols infinitely more frequently than the healthy: that is, they employ symbols without any regard for their appropriateness in the given situation.[10]

Bleuler's explanation of these symptoms creates fresh problems for the psychiatrist, logician, humanist, and civil libertarian. For this now-classic psychiatric perspective presses these questions upon us: If what makes schizophrenic utterances symptoms is that they are incomprehensible, do they still remain symptoms after they are no longer incomprehensible? If the utterances are comprehensible, why confine those who utter them in madhouses? Indeed, why confine

9. Ibid., p. 151.
10. Ibid., p. 428.

persons even if their utterances are incomprehensible? These are the questions Bleuler never asks. Moreover, they are the questions that cannot be raised in psychiatry even today, for such queries expose the empires of psychiatry as being as devoid of visible diseases as a well-known emperor was of visible clothes.

Consider in this connection the woman patient who, Bleuler writes, " 'possesses' Switzerland; and in the same sense she says, 'I am Switzerland.' She may also say, 'I am freedom,' since for her Switzerland meant nothing less than freedom." According to Bleuler,

> The difference between the use of such phrases in the healthy and in the schizophrenics rests in the fact that in the former it is a mere metaphor, whereas for the patients the dividing line between direct and indirect representation has been obscured. The result is that they frequently think of these metaphors in a literal sense.[11]

The source of Bleuler's egocentric and ethnocentric fallacy is dramatically evident here. Would a Catholic psychiatrist writing in a Catholic country have expressed himself so cavalierly about the literalization of metaphor constituting the cardinal symptom of schizophrenia, the most malignant form of madness known to medical science? For what, from a Protestant point of view, is the Catholic doctrine of transubstantiation if not the literalization of a metaphor? *Mutatis mutandis*, I have argued that the psychiatric conception of mental illness is also a literalized metaphor.[12] The main difference in my view between these cardinal Catholic and psychiatric metaphors and the metaphors of so-called schizophrenic patients lies not in any linguistic or logical peculiarity of the respective symbols, but in their social legitimacy.

The main purpose of my foregoing remarks was to show that our intuitive judgment about other people's humanity made on the basis of whether they express themselves as we do is untrustworthy. Hence, this criterion of humanness must be repudiated by humanists. The change could, I think, be salutary: it might lead to a perspective on people at least as humane as is our perspective on animals and

11. Ibid., p. 429.

12. *The Myth of Mental Illness: Foundations of a Theory of Personal Conduct*, rev. ed. (New York: Harper & Row, 1974), and "Mental Illness as a Metaphor," *Nature* 242 (March 1973): 305–307.

things. We do not demand that bees explain to us the language of insects or that Egyptian tablets explain to us the meaning of hieroglyphics, and we do not conclude that unless they can explain their languages to our satisfaction, they are incomprehensible or meaningless. Yet that is exactly what psychiatrists—and to a large extent everyone else—have done with respect to so-called mental patients: they insist that the patient give them an account of himself satisfactory to them—and if the patient fails to do so, they declare him to be ill and imprison him as insane.

Why do we not expect the same intellectual responsibility from ourselves when we face the riddle that the behavior of other people poses for us as we do when we face the riddle that the behavior of animals and things poses for us? Formerly, persons whose behavior was regarded as incomprehensibly wicked were called heretics and witches; now they are called mental patients. Who knows what they will be called tomorrow? Obviously, these behaviors are wicked only because they violate the core values of those in power, and they are incomprehensible only because those who ostensibly try to understand them in fact try not to and define them as incomprehensible and hence irrational.

In this connection, I would like to mention a paradox that has long struck me as bitterly ironic. In the field of animal behavior—now a large and growing discipline—workers often compare the communicative behavior of porpoises to those of people and call their signaling behavior language. In the earlier days of psychiatry—when the keepers of madmen were more correctly called mad-doctors and alienists—the keepers compared madmen to wild beasts and viewed the pleas of the insane as the squeals of caged animals. Today—when the keepers are medical scientists—psychiatrists compare the schizophrenic to the syphilitic and view his thought disorder as a manifestation of his brain disorder. The ethologist may thus be said to have a burning passion for humanizing animals and the psychiatrist for dehumanizing persons.

My foregoing remarks are pertinent to the concerns of humanists not only because they throw fresh light on the relations between how people use language and how other people judge them, as more or less sane, or more or less human, but also because they throw fresh light on the dual function of language, especially in human relations—that is, for understanding people and for controlling them. This dual function of language in human relations stands in sharp contrast to the singular function of language in relation to animals and things: in our relations with the nonhuman world, we use language only for understanding and employ some sort of direct—nonverbal, nonsymbolic—action for control.[13] The upshot is that we often claim that we want to understand another person when in fact we want to control him. Indeed, it is when we most want to control others that we usually make two contradictory claims about them—namely, that their behavior is incomprehensible and that we understand their behavior better than they understand it themselves. We should be skeptical of such claims whether they are offered by psychiatrists or psychologists, psychoanalysts or psychohistorians—our newest breed of psychoassassins, who, of course, consider themselves to be our humanists *par excellence*. Faced with such explanations and explainers, we should ask, *Cui bono?* Who benefits from such explanations? What is the relationship between subject and explainer? Are they friends or foes? Does the subject want to be an object of explanation at all? For it is obvious that explaining a person's behavior against his will, and explaining it when one holds him in contempt, is, albeit ostensibly an explanation, actually a metaphorical confinement: such an explanation confines by means of a contemptuous and degrading imagery, just as banishment, prison, and the gallows confine by means of degrading and destructive action.

The struggle for human liberty and dignity is now being waged on many fronts and in many different ways. As humanists—as linguistic humanists, if I may suggest a tentative self-description some of us might find fitting—we could, and should, be in the vanguard of those whose weapons are pens, not swords; typewriters and books, not demonstrations and bombs. That means that we must defend human rights because the victims are human beings. If you find that assertion contrived or opaque, may I remind you that it is currently popular for humanists and civil libertarians to champion

13. See my *Ideology and Insanity: Essays on the Psychiatric Dehumanization of Man* (Garden City, N.Y.: Doubleday, Anchor Press, 1970), pp. 190–217.

the "rights of the mentally ill" and the rights of other victimized groups such as homosexuals, drug addicts, blacks, women, and so forth. From the point of view I am trying to articulate, all that is a grave mistake. We should reject slogans such as "protecting the rights of the mentally ill" (and of other victimized groups); instead, we should protect the rights of people to reject being called or categorized as mentally ill (or anything else) against their will (except as part of the process of the administration of the criminal law). In other words, we should stand steadfast for the right of men and women to reject those involuntary identifications or diagnoses that have traditionally justified and made possible, and often continue to justify and make possible, their inferior or subhuman treatment at the hands of those who ostensibly care for them but who actually scapegoat them.

Specifically, we should insist that the members of certain victimized groups have no right to treatment, to abortion or day-care centers, to methadone, or to any other service or special consideration; what they do have a right to, however, is to be considered and called persons or human beings. Moreover, as there are no rights without corresponding duties, this position—in contrast to the currently popular paternalistic-therapeutic position toward the insane, the poor, women, and so forth—implies, first, that, however different certain members of these groups might be from us, we should refuse to regard them as a priori better or worse, more or less deserving, than anyone else in society; and, second, that these victims should accept the same obligation of regarding themselves as neither inherently better than or superior to, nor worse than or inferior to, others. We cannot have our cake and eat it too; we cannot preach humanism and practice male or female chauvinism, paternalism, or therapeutism.

In concluding, I should like to return to my original proposition that high among the humanist's concerns should be language and, in particular, his own disciplined use of it. That this is not a novel idea I not only acknowledge but emphasize. I respect intellectual tradition too highly to believe that a humanist should even aspire to novelty. I believe that, instead, he should try to reaffirm and rearticulate the wisdom of the humanists who have gone before him and should build on the solid, albeit familiar, foundation that they have laid down for us.

Accordingly, I should like to end by citing some observations on language that best express those timeless principles and practices to which, as humanists, we must perpetually recommit ourselves.

"A Chinese sage of the distant past," as Erich Heller tells it,

> was once asked by his disciples what he would do first if he were given power to set right the affairs of the country. He answered: "I should certainly see to it that language is used correctly." The disciples looked perplexed. "Surely," they said, "this is a trivial matter. Why should you deem it so important?" And the Master replied: "If language is not used correctly, then what is said is not what is meant; if what is said is not what is meant, then what ought to be done remains undone; if this remains undone, morals and art will be corrupted; if morals and art are corrupted, justice will go astray; if justice goes astray, the people will stand about in helpless confusion."[14]

In our own day, George Orwell was obsessed—in the loftiest sense of this word—by the idea that language was the very soul of man. "Newspeak" is not a warning about an imaginary, future threat to human dignity; it is the imaginative rendering of an ancient, perhaps perennial, human proclivity to corrupt and control man by corrupting and controlling his language. Orwell's short essay "Politics and the English Language" may well serve as a manifesto for linguistic humanists. In it, he writes:

> The inflated style is itself a kind of euphemism. A mass of Latin words falls upon facts like soft snow, blurring the outlines and covering up all the details. The great enemy of clear language is insincerity. When there is a gap between one's real and one's declared aims, one turns as it were instinctively to long words and exhausted idioms, like a cuttlefish squirting out ink. In our age there is no such thing as "keeping out of politics." All issues are political issues, and politics itself is a mass of lies, evasions, folly, hatred, and schizophrenia. When the general atmosphere is bad, language must suffer. I should expect to find—this is a guess which I have not sufficient knowledge to verify—

14. E. Heller, "A Symposium: Assessment of the Man and the Philospher," in K. T. Fann, ed., *Ludwig Wittgenstein: The Man and His Philosophy* (New York: Dell, Delta Books, 1967), p. 64.

that the German, Russian, Italian languages have all deteriorated in the last ten or fifteen years, as a result of dictatorship.[15]

Orwell concludes with a recommendation we might well adopt as our credo:

> . . . one ought to recognize that the present political chaos is connected with the decay of language, and that one can probably bring about some improvement by starting at the verbal end. If you simplify your English, you are freed from the worst follies of orthodoxy. You cannot speak any of the necessary dialects, and when you make a stupid remark its stupidity will be obvious, even to yourself. Political language . . . is designed to make lies sound truthful and murder respectable, and to give an appearance of solidity to pure wind. One cannot change this all in a moment, but one can at least change one's own habits.[16]

Everything Orwell says here about political language applies also, perhaps with even greater force, to the languages of the so-called behavioral sciences and, among them, especially to that of psychiatry. Yet it is to behavioral scientists, and especially to psychiatrists—who call and consider themselves humanists and are generally so considered by others—that the modern humanist movement has often looked for inspiration and guidance. That is a grievous error: among the enemies of humanism, psychiatry—that is to say, the ideology of mental health and mental illness and the psychiatric deceptions and coercions justified in its name—is one of the most dangerous and most powerful. Terence, we might here recall, said, "I am a man, nothing human is alien to me." The psychiatrist has inverted that. He declares, "I am a psychiatrist, nothing alien is human to me," thus reasserting the old, barbaric view of the human.

Recognizing an adversary concealed as an ally, unmasking a foe masquerading as a friend, is, however, half the battle. As for the rest of it—the battle against one of the most vicious contemporary sociopolitical creeds that wages war against human freedom and

15. G. Orwell, "Politics and the English Language," in *The Orwell Reader: Fiction, Essays, and Reportage* (New York: Harcourt Brace Jovanovich, 1956), pp. 363–364.
16. Ibid., p. 366.

dignity by corrupting language—everything, or very nearly everything, remains to be done. I am confident, however, that if we succeed in this struggle—or, better, in proportion as we succeed in it—it will be not because we are reasonable or well-meaning, rational or liberal, religious or secular, but rather because we protect and perfect our souls by protecting and perfecting our language.

# 8

# The Right to Health

In every society—whether it be tribal or industrial, theological or secular, capitalist or Communist—goods and services are distributed unequally. That is, in fact, what the words *rich* and *poor* really mean; it is their "operational definition": the rich have, and the poor have not. The "haves" eat more nutritious foods, dwell in more comfortable and spacious homes, and travel by means of more luxurious transportation than do the "have nots." Similar differences exist between the same persons and groups with respect to medical care. When the rich man falls ill, he occupies a hospital bed in a single room or private suite and receives treatment from the best—or at least the most expensive—physicians in town. When the poor man falls ill, he occupies a bed in the charity ward—though it may no longer be called that—and receives treatment from young men who, though called *doctor*, are only medical students. In short, though it is not a disgrace to be poor, it is not a great honor either.

Although it is self-evident that the poor will always have more needs than the rich and the rich more satisfactions than the poor, that fact is now repeatedly discovered and denounced by psychiatric epidemiologists. For example, Ernest Gruenberg declares that there is in our society "a pattern in which the prevalence of illness is an inverse function of family income, while the volume of medical care received is a direct function of family income."[1] In plain English,

1. E. Gruenberg, "Counting Sick People," *Science* 161 (July 1968): 347.

that means that poverty begets sickness and affluence begets medical attention. The same statement, of course, could be made about every other important human need and satisfaction. For example, to earn a living, a poor man has a greater need for transportation than does a rich man, who could stay at home and live off his investments; yet the former must do with the inferior public transportation system provided by the community whereas the latter enjoys a fleet of private cars, boats, and airplanes. Such considerations do not deter Gruenberg, and many other physicians addressing themselves to the subject, from observing—plaintively and, I think, rather naïvely—that "one may doubt . . . [that] efforts to redistribute medical care have eliminated the paradox."[2] But there is no paradox—except, that is, in the eyes of the utopian social reformer who views all social differences as contagious diseases waiting to be wiped out by his therapeutic efforts.

The concept that medical treatment is a right rather than a privilege has gained increasing support during the past decade.[3] The advocates of the concept are no doubt motivated by good intentions: they wish to correct certain inequalities in the distribution of health services in American society. That such inequalities exist is not in dispute. What is in dispute, however, is how to distinguish between inequalities and inequities and how to determine which governmental policies are best suited to the securing of good medical care for the maximum number of persons.[4]

The desire to improve the lot of less fortunate people is laudable; indeed, I share that desire. Still, unless all inequalities are considered to be inequities—a view clearly incompatible with social

2. Ibid.

3. See, for example, B. S. Brown, "Psychiatric Practice and Public Policy," *American Journal of Psychiatry* 125 (August 1968): 141–146.

4. Ever since the French Revolution, and increasingly during the past century, virtually all Western governments have fostered the belief that not only great inequalities of wealth but inequalities of all kinds—for example, of ambition, of talent, and of course of health—are inequities. The result has been described with unmatched irony by C. S. Lewis: "Men are not angered by mere misfortune, but by misfortune conceived as injury. And the sense of injury depends on the feeling that a legitimate claim has been denied. The more claims on life, therefore, that your patient can be induced to make, the more often he will feel injured" (*The Screwtape Letters and Screwtape Proposes a Toast* [New York: Macmillan, 1971], pp. 95–96).

organization and human life as we know it—two important questions remain: First, which inequalities should be considered inequities? Second, what are the most appropriate means for minimizing or abolishing the inequalities we deem unjust? Appeals to good intentions are of no help in answering those questions.

There are two groups of people whose situation with respect to medical care the advocates of the concept of a right to treatment regard as especially unfair or unjust and whose condition they seek to ameliorate. One group is composed of poor people who need ordinary medical care. The other group is composed of the inmates of the public mental hospitals who supposedly need psychiatric care. However, the propositions that poor people ought to have access to more, better, or less expensive medical care than they do now and that people in public mental hospitals ought to receive better psychiatric care than they do now pose two quite different problems. I shall therefore deal with each separately.

The availability of medical services for a particular person, or group of persons, in a particular society depends principally on the supply of the desired services and the prospective user's powers to command those services. No government or organization—whether it be the United States government, the American Medical Association, or the Communist Party of the Soviet Union—can provide medical care except insofar as it has the power to control the education of physicians, their right to practice medicine, and the manner in which they dispose of their time and energies. In other words, only individuals can provide medical treatment for sick people; institutions, such as the church and the state, can promote, permit, or prohibit certain therapeutic activities but cannot by themselves provide medical services.

Social groups wielding power are notoriously prone to prohibit the free exercise of certain human skills and the availability of certain drugs and devices. For example, during the declining Middle Ages and the early Renaissance period, the Church repeatedly prohibited Jewish physicians from practicing medicine and non-Jewish patients from seeking their services. The same prohibition was imposed by the state in Nazi Germany. In the modern democracies of the free West, the state continues to exercise its prerogative to prohibit certain kinds of therapeutic activities. To be sure, the prohibition is no longer based on the ground that the healers have the wrong religion; instead, it is now based on the ground that they are untrained or inadequately trained as physicians. This situation is an inevitable consequence of the fact that the state's licensing powers fulfill two unrelated and mutually incompatible functions: to protect the public—that is, the actual or potential patients—from incompetent medical practitioners by insuring an adequate level of training and competence on the part of all physicians, and to protect the members of a special vested-interest group—that is, the physicians—from competition from an excessive number of similarly trained practitioners and from healers of different persuasions and skills who might prove more useful to their would-be clients than those officially approved. The result is a complex and powerful alliance, first, between the church and medicine and, subsequently, between the state and medicine—with physicians playing double roles as medical healers and as agents of social control. The restrictive function of the state with respect to medical practice has been, and continues to be, especially significant in the United States.

Without delving further into the intricacies of this large and complex subject, it should suffice to note that our present system of medical training and practice is far removed from that of laissez faire capitalism for which many, and especially its opponents, mistake it. In actuality, the American Medical Association is not only an immensely powerful lobby of medical vested interests, but a force that the reformers ardently support.[5] The consequence of the alliance between organized medicine and the American government has been the creation of a system of education and licensure with tight controls over the production and distribution of health care in a context of an artificially created chronic shortage of medical personnel. That result has been achieved by limiting the number of practitioners through the regulation of medical licensure.

The laws of economics being what they are, when the supply of a given service is smaller than the demand for it we have a seller's market; that is good for the sellers, in this case the medical profession. Conversely, when the supply is greater than the demand, we

5. See, for example, J. S. Clark, Jr., "Can the Liberals Rally?" *Atlantic Monthly*, July 1953, pp. 27–31.

have a buyer's market; that is good for the buyers, in this case the potential patients. One way—and according to the supporters of a free-market economy, the best way—to help buyers get more of what they want at the lowest possible price is to increase the supply of the needed product or service. That would suggest that instead of government grants for special neighborhood health centers and community mental-health centers, the medical needs of the less affluent members of American society could be better served simply by repealing laws governing medical licensure.[6] As logical as that may seem, in medical and liberal circles, this suggestion is regarded as hare-brained or worse.

Since medical care in the United States is in short supply, its availability to the poor may be improved by redistributing the existing supply, by increasing the supply, or by both. Many individuals and groups clamoring for an improvement in our medical-care system fail to scrutinize the artificially created shortage of medical personnel and refuse to look to the free market for a restoration of the balance between demand and supply. Instead, they seek to remedy the imbalance by redistributing the existing supply —in effect, robbing Peter to pay Paul. That proposal is in the tradition of other modern liberal social reforms, such as the redistribution of wealth by progressive taxation and a system of compulsory social security. No doubt, a political and economic system more

6. The deleterious effects on the public of professional licensure in general, and of medical licensure in particular, have been well analyzed and articulated by Milton Friedman. He notes that the justification for enacting special licensure provisons, especially for regulating medical practice, "is always said to be the necessity of protecting the public interest. However, the pressure on the legislature to license an occupation rarely comes from the members of the public. . . . On the contrary, the pressure invariably comes from members of the occupation itself" (*Capitalism and Freedom* [Chicago: University of Chicago Press, 1962], p. 140).

Unless one believes in the special altruism of physicians (for which there is no evidence), the conclusion is inescapable that the actual aim of restrictive licensure laws—as contrasted with the certification of the special competence of such people as mathematicians or physicists, which carries no implication of legal restraints on others not so certified—is the very opposite of their ostensible or professed aim. Under the pretense of protecting the public from incompetent practitioners, they protect the profession from the competition of other vendors of desired services and from the scrutiny of an enlightened public.

socialistic in character than the one we now have could promote an equalization in the quality of the medical care received by the rich and the poor. Whether that would result in the quality of the medical care of the poor approximating that of the rich or vice versa would remain to be seen. Experience surely suggests the latter. For over a century, we have had our version of state-supported psychiatric care for all who need it—namely, the state mental-hospital system. The results of that effort are available for all to see.

Ironically, it is precisely the inadequacy of care in public mental institutions that has inspired the concept of a right to treatment. In two landmark decisions handed down by the U.S. Court of Appeals for the District of Columbia Circuit, the court affirmed the concept of a right to treatment for persons confined in public mental hospitals. In *Rouse* v. *Cameron*, Judge Bazelon, speaking for the majority, declared that "the purpose of involuntary hospitalization is treatment, not punishment"; noted that "Congress established a *statutory* 'right to treatment' in the 1964 Hospitalization of the Mentally Ill Act"; and concluded that "the patient's right to treatment is clear."[7]

It might be noted that Rouse had been involuntarily committed to Saint Elizabeth's Hospital in November 1962 after a finding of not guilty by reason of insanity of carrying a dangerous weapon. Had Rouse been found guilty of that offense, the maximum sentence would have been one year in prison. However, having been "acquitted," he had at the time of his appeal already spent four years in Saint Elizabeth's Hospital. Moreover, Rouse contended that he had never been mentally ill, that he was not mentally ill, and that he never needed psychiatric treatment—opinions that Bazelon not only ignored but inverted into their very opposites.

On the day the Rouse decision was handed down, the same court reiterated and extended its views on the right to treatment in *Millard* v. *Cameron*. Millard had been charged with indecent exposure in June 1962, pleaded guilty to the charge, and was subsequently committed to Saint Elizabeth's Hospital as a "sexual psychopath." His appeal was based on the contention that he was

7. *Rouse* v. *Cameron*, 125 U.S. App. D.C. 366, 373 F. 2d 451 (1966), pp. 452, 453, 456.

receiving no treatment. Judge Bazelon, again speaking for the court, declared: "In *Rouse* v. *Cameron* . . . [we] held that the petitioner was entitled to relief upon showing that he was not receiving reasonably suited and adequate treatment. Lack of such treatment, we said, could not be justified by lack of staff or facilities. We think the same principles apply to a person involuntarily committed to a public hospital as a sexual psychopath."[8]

However, in neither *Rouse* nor *Millard* did Judge Bazelon define what "adequate treatment" was or say what, in the court's opinion, would constitute clearly inadequate treatment. Let us therefore examine what the concept of a right to medical or psychiatric treatment entails and implies.[9]

Most people in public mental hospitals do not receive what one would ordinarily consider treatment. With that as his starting point, Morton Birnbaum has advocated "the recognition and enforcement of the legal right of a mentally ill inmate of a public mental institution to adequate medical treatment for his mental illness."[10] Although it defined neither "mental illness" nor "adequate medical treatment," the proposal was received with enthusiasm in both legal and medical circles.[11] Why? Because it supported the myth that mental illness is a medical problem that can be solved by medical means.

The idea of a *right* to mental treatment is both naïve and dangerous. It is naïve because it considers the problem of the publicly hospitalized mental patient as medical, rather than educational, economic, religious, and social. It is dangerous because the proposed remedy creates another problem—compulsory mental treatment—for, in the context of involuntary confinement, the treatment too must be compulsory.

8. *Millard* v. *Cameron*, 125 U.S. App. D.C. 383, 373 F. 2d 468 (1966), p. 472.

9. In this connection, see my *Law, Liberty, and Psychiatry: An Inquiry into the Social Uses of Mental Health Practices* (New York: Macmillan, 1963), pp. 214–216.

10. M. Birnbaum, "The Right to Treatment," *American Bar Association Journal* 46 (1960): 499.

11. See, for example, T. Gregory, "A New Right" (editorial), *American Bar Association Journal* (1960): 516; and *The New York Times*, December 15, 1967.

Hailing the right to treatment as a "new right," the editor of the *American Bar Association Journal* compared psychiatric treatment for patients in public mental hospitals with monetary compensation for the unemployed. In both cases, we are told, the principle is to help the "victims of unfortunate circumstances."[12]

But things are not so simple. We know what unemployment is; but we are not so clear about what mental illness is. Moreover, a person without a job does not usually object to receiving money, and if he does, no one compels him to take it. The situation of the involuntarily hospitalized mental patient is quite different; he does not want psychiatric treatment, and the more he objects to it, the more firmly society insists that he must have it.

Of course, if we define psychiatric treatment as *help for the victims of unfortunate circumstances*, how can anyone object to it? But the real question is twofold: What is meant by psychiatric help? and What should the helpers do if the victim refuses to be helped?

From a legal and sociological point of view, the only way to define mental illness is to enumerate the types of behavior psychiatrists consider indicative of such illness. Similarly, we may define psychiatric treatment by listing the procedures that psychiatrists regard as instances of such therapy. A brief illustration should suffice.

Maurice Levine lists forty methods of psychotherapy. Among them, he includes physical treatment, medicinal treatment, reassurance, authoritative firmness, hospitalization, ignoring of certain symptoms and attitudes, satisfaction of neurotic needs, and bibliotherapy. In addition, there are physical methods of psychiatric therapy, such as the prescription of sedatives and tranquilizers, the induction of convulsions by drugs or electricity, and brain surgery.[13] Obviously, the term *psychiatric treatment* covers everything that may be done to a person under medical auspices—and more.

If psychiatric treatment is all the things Levine and others tell us it is, how are we to determine whether or not patients in mental hospitals receive adequate amounts of it? Surely, many of them are already being treated with large doses of authoritative firmness, with ignoring of symptoms, and certainly with satisfaction of neurotic

12. Gregory, "A New Right ," p. 516.
13. M. Levine, *Psychotherapy in Medical Practice* (New York: Macmillan, 1942), pp. 17–18.

needs. This last therapeutic agent has particularly sinister possibilities for offenders. Psychoanalysts have long maintained that many criminals commit antisocial acts out of a sense of guilt. What they neurotically crave is punishment. By that logic, indefinite incarceration itself might be regarded as psychiatric treatment.

At present, our publicly operated psychiatric institutions perform their services on the premise that it is morally legitimate to treat so-called mentally sick persons against their will. Illustrative is a document prepared by the Committee on the Recodification of the New York State Mental Hygiene Law. It begins with the declaration that "it is axiomatic that the entire Mental Hygiene Law is concerned with patients' rights, especially rights to adequate care and treatment."[14]

That assertion is a brazen falsehood. The primary concern of any mental-hygiene law is to empower physicians to imprison innocent citizens under the rubric of "civil commitment" and to justify torturing them by means of a variety of violent acts called *psychiatric treatments*. As one would expect, among the members of the above-mentioned committee were the commissioner and two assistant commissioners of the New York State Department of Mental Hygiene. Conspicuous by their absence from the committee were inmates of public mental hospitals, or former inmates, or experts selected by these "patients" to represent them.

In relation to psychiatric treatment, then, the most fundamental and vexing problem is this: how can a treatment that is compulsory also be a right? As I have shown elsewhere, the problem posed by the mistreatment of the publicly hospitalized mentally ill derives not from any insufficiency in the treatment they receive, but rather from the basic conceptual fallacy inherent in the notion of mental illness and from the moral evil inherent in the practice of involuntary mental hospitalization.[15] Preserving the concept of mental illness and the social practices it has justified and papering over its glaring cognitive and ethical defects by means of a superimposed right to mental treatment only aggravates an already intolerably oppressive situation.

14. Institute of Public Administration, "A Mental Hygiene Law for New York State," Art. 37, February 1968 draft.

15. *Law, Liberty, and Psychiatry.*

The problem posed by the "warehousing" of vast numbers of unwanted, helpless, and stigmatized people in huge state mental hospitals could be better resolved—better, that is, for the victimized patients, though not necessarily for the society that is victimizing them or for the professionals who profit from this arrangement—by asking, What do involuntarily hospitalized mental patients need more—a right to receive treatments they do not want or a right to refuse such interventions?

As my foregoing remarks indicate, I see two fundamental defects in the concept of a right to treatment. One is scientific and medical, stemming from unclarified issues concerning what constitutes an illness or a treatment and who qualifies as a patient or physician. The other is political and moral, stemming from unclarified issues concerning the differences between rights and claims.

In the present state of medical practice and popular opinion, the definitions of the terms *illness*, *treatment*, *physician*, and *patient* are so imprecise that the concept of a right to treatment can only serve to muddy further an already extremely confused situation. For example, one can treat, in the medical sense of the term, only a disease or, more precisely, only a person, now called a patient, suffering from a disease. But what is a disease? Certainly, cancer, stroke, and heart disease are. But is obesity a disease? How about smoking cigarettes? Using heroin or marijuana? Malingering to avoid the draft or collect insurance compensation? Homosexuality? Kleptomania? Grief? Each of those conditions has been declared a disease by medical and psychiatric authorities who hold impeccable institutional credentials. And so have innumerable other conditions from bachelorhood, divorce, and unwanted pregnancy to political and religious prejudice.

Similarly, what is treatment? Certainly, the surgical removal of a cancerous breast is. But is an organ transplant treatment? If it is and if such a treatment is a right, how can those charged with guaranteeing people the protection of their right to treatment discharge their duties without having acess to the requisite number of transplantable organs? On a simpler level, if ordinary obesity, due to eating too much, is a disease, how can a doctor treat it when its treatment depends on the patient eating less? What does it mean then that a patient has a right to be treated for obesity? I have already alluded to how easily that kind of right becomes equated with a societal and medical obligation to deprive the patient of his freedom—to eat, to drink, to take drugs, and so forth.

Furthermore, who is a patient? Is he someone who has a demonstrable bodily illness or injury—such as cancer or a fracture? A person who complains of bodily symptoms but has no demonstrable illness, like the so-called hypochondriac? The person who feels perfectly well but is said to be ill by others, like the so-called paranoid schizophrenic? Or is he a person who professes political views differing from those of the psychiatrists who brand him insane, like Senator Barry Goldwater?

Finally, who is a physician? Is he a person licensed to practice medicine? One certified to have completed a specified educational curriculum? One possessing certain medical skills as demonstrated by public performance? Or is he one claiming to possess such skills?

It seems to me that improvements in the medical care of poor people and in the care of people now said to be mentally ill depend less on declarations about their rights to treatment than on certain reforms in the speech and conduct of those professing a desire to help them. In particular, such reforms would have to entail refinements in the use of such medical concepts as illness and treatment and a recognition of the basic differences between medical intervention as a service, which the individual is free to seek or reject, and medical intervention as a method of social control, which is imposed on him by force or fraud.

I can perhaps best illustrate the unsolved dilemmas of what constitute diseases and treatment by citing some actual cases. As recently as 1965, a Connecticut statute made it a crime for any person to artificially prevent conception.[16] Accordingly, a mother

16. In *Griswold* v. *Connecticut*, the Connecticut anticontraceptive statute was declared unconstitutional by the Supreme Court on the ground that it violated the right of marital privacy, a right the court considered within the penumbra of the specific guarantees of the Bill of Rights. The significance of this case lies in its offering an instance in which a state's duly appointed legislators denied a certain kind of medical assistance to their constituents, while a majority of the Supreme Court deemed such assistance a right. Connecticut General Statutes Revised, § 53–32 (Supp. 1965), ruled invalid in *Griswold* v. *Connecticut*, 381 U.S. 479 (1965).

of ten requesting contraceptive help from a physician in a public hospital in Connecticut would have been refused such assistance. Did what she seek constitute treatment? Not according to the legislators who defined the prescription of birth-control devices as immoral and illegal acts rather than as interventions aimed at preserving health.

Today, a similar situation obtains with respect to a woman's unwanted pregnancy and her wish for an abortion. Is being pregnant when one does not want to be an illness? Is abortion a treatment, or is it the murder of a fetus? If it is murder, why is no abortionist ever prosecuted for *murder*? How can the preservation of a pregnant woman's mental health justify such killing, now called *therapeutic abortion*?[17]

On the other hand, should a wholly secular, utilitarian point of view prevail and the use of birth-control devices and abortion be considered treatments, what would it mean for a woman to have a right to such interventions? Clearly, it would have to mean that she has a right to unhampered access to physicians willing to prescribe birth-control devices and perform abortions. Where would such a medico-legal posture leave a Roman Catholic obstetrician? By refusing to abort a woman wishing a termination of her pregnancy, he would be interfering with her right to treatment in a way that might be analogized to a white barber's refusal to cut the hair of a black customer, or vice versa, thus interfering with his customer's civil rights.

As still another example, consider the situation of an unhappily married couple. Are they sick? If they define themselves as neurotic and consult a psychiatrist, they are considered sick and their insurance coverage may even pay for their treatment. But if they seek the solution of their problem in divorce and consult an attorney, they are not considered sick. Thus, although unhappily married people are often considered ill, divorce is never considered to be a treatment. If it were, it too would have to be a right. Where would that leave our present divorce laws?

One could go on and on. I shall cite, however, only one more

17. In this connection, see my "The Ethics of Birth Control," *The Humanist* 20 (November–December 1960): 332–336, and "The Ethics of Abortion," ibid., 26 (September–October 1966): 147–148.

instance—the practice of involuntary mental hospitalization—to show how deeply confused and confusing is our present situation with respect to the concept of treatment and hence how very mischievous any extension of the concept of a right to treatment, as a right secured by the government, is bound to be.

In most jurisdictions, persons said to be mentally ill and dangerous to themselves or others may be committed to a mental hospital. Such incarceration in a building called a hospital is considered a form of psychiatric, and hence medical, treatment. But who in fact is the patient? Who is being treated? Ostensibly, the person treated is the one who is incarcerated. But since he does not seek medical help, whereas those who secure his confinement do, one might argue that involuntary mental hospitalization is treatment for those who seek commitment rather than for those who are committed. That would be analogous to arguing that a therapeutic abortion is treatment for the pregnant woman, not for the aborted fetus—an assertion few would deny. If that argument is accepted, in any conflict injuring one party could be defined as a treatment of his opponent. The following recent statement on the psychiatric treatment of "acting-out adolescents" is illustrative: "The move toward 'freedom, love, peace,' has encouraged anti-social acting out, including the increasing use of marijuana and psychedelic drugs. Consequently, emotionally disturbed young men who are acting in a way that directly conflicts with their parents' standards are being hospitalized in increasing numbers."[18] In that sort of situation, whose right to treatment do the advocates of such hospitalization wish to guarantee —that of the parent to commit his rebellious child as mentally ill or that of the child to defy his parents without being subjected to quasi-medical penalties?

The second difficulty posed by the concept of a right to treatment is of a political and moral nature. It stems from confusing rights with claims and protection from injuries with provision of goods or services.

18. L. W. Krinsky and R. M. Jennings, "The Management and Treatment of Acting-Out Adolescents in a Separate Unit," *Hospital and Community Psychiatry* 19 (March 1968): 72.

For a definition of *right*, I can do no better than to quote John Stuart Mill. In *Utilitarianism*, he writes:

> I have treated the idea of a right as *residing in the injured person and violated by the injury*. . . . When we call anything a person's right we mean that he has a valid claim on society to protect him in the possession of it, either by the force of law, or by that of education and opinion. . . . To have a right, then, is, I conceive, to have something which *society ought to defend me in the possession of*. [Italics added.][19]

Mill's distinction helps us to distinguish rights from claims. Rights, Mill says, are "possessions"; they are things people have by nature, like liberty; acquire by dint of hard work, like property; create by inventiveness, like a new machine; or inherit, like money. Characteristically, possessions are what a person *has*, and of which others, including the state, can therefore deprive him. Mill's point is the classic libertarian one—the state ought to protect the individual in his rights. That is what the Declaration of Independence means when it refers to the inalienable rights to life, liberty, and the pursuit of happiness. It is important to note that, in political theory no less than in everyday practice, that requires that the state be strong and resolute enough to protect the rights of the individual from infringement by others and that it be decentralized and restrained enough, typically through federalism and a constitution, to insure that it will not itself violate the rights of the people.

In the sense specified above, then, there can be no such thing as a right to treatment. Conceiving of a person's body as his possession—like his automobile or watch (though no doubt more valuable)—it is just as nonsensical to speak of his right to have his body repaired as it would be to speak of his right to have his automobile or watch repaired.

It is thus evident that in its current usage, and especially in the phrase *right to treatment*, the term *right* actually means *claim*. More specifically, *right* here means the recognition of the claims of one party, considered to be *in the right*, and the repudiation of the claims of another, opposing party, considered to be *in the wrong*

19. J. S. Mill, *Utilitarianism*, in M. Lerner, ed., *Essential Works of John Stuart Mill* (New York: Bantam Books, 1961), p. 238.

—the rightful party having allied himself with the interests of the community and enlisted the coercive powers of the state on his own behalf. Let us analyze that situation in the case of medical treatment for ordinary bodily disease—for example, diabetes. The patient, having lost some of his health, tries to regain it by means of medical attention and drugs. The medical attention he needs is, however, the property of the physician, and the drug he needs is the property of the manufacturer who produced it. The patient's right to treatment thus conflicts, first, with the physician's right to liberty—that is, to sell his services freely—and, second, with the pharmaceutical manufacturer's right to property—that is, to sell his products as he chooses. The advocates of a right to treatment for the patient are less than candid regarding their proposals for reconciling that alleged right with the actual rights of the physician to liberty and of the pharmaceutical manufacturer to property.

Nor is it clear how the concept of a right to treatment can be reconciled with the traditional Western concept of the patient's right to choose his physician. If the patient has a right to choose the doctor by whom he wishes to be treated and if he also has a right to treatment, then in effect the doctor is the patient's slave. Obviously, the patient's right to choose his physician cannot be wrenched from its context and survive: its corollary is the physician's right to accept or reject a patient (except for rare cases of emergency treatment). No one of course envisions the absurdity of physicians being at the personal beck and call of individual patients, becoming literally their medical slaves as some had been in ancient Greece and Rome.

The concept of a right to treatment has a different, much less absurd but far more ominous, implication. For just as the corollary of the individual's freedom to choose his physician is the physician's freedom to refuse treating any particular patient, so the corollary of the individual's right to treatment is the denial of the physician's right to reject as a patient anyone officially so designated. The transformation of the medical relationship, from individualistic and contractural to bureaucratic and coercive, in one fell swoop removes the individual's right to define himself as sick and to seek medical care as he sees fit and the physician's right to define whom he considers to be sick and wishes to treat; it places those decisions instead in the hands of the state's medical bureaucracy. To see how that works in the United States and on a less-than-total scale, coexisting with a flourishing system of private medical practice, one need only look at our state mental hospitals. Every patient admitted to such a hospital has a right to treatment, and every physician serving in such a hospital system has an obligation to treat any patient assigned to him by his superiors or committed to his care by the courts. Missing from the system, and similar systems, are the patient's traditional economic and legal controls over the medical relationship and the physician's traditional economic dependence on, and legal obligations to, the individual he has accepted as a patient.

As a result, bureaucratic, as contrasted with entrepreneurial, medical care ceases to be a system of curing disease and becomes instead a system of controlling deviance. Although that outcome seems to me inevitable in the case of psychiatry (in view of the fact that ascription of the label *mental illness* usually functions as quasi-medical rhetoric concealing social conflicts), it need not be inevitable for nonpsychiatric medical services. However, in every situation where medical care is provided bureaucratically (as in Communist societies), the physician's role as agent of the sick patient is necessarily alloyed with, and often seriously compromised by, his role as agent of the state. Thus, the doctor becomes a kind of medical policeman, sometimes helping the individual and sometimes harming him.

Returning to Mill's definition of a right, one could say further that just as a man has a right to life and liberty, so too has he a right to health and hence a claim on the state to protect his health. It is important to note here that the right to health differs from the right to treatment in the same way as the right to property differs from the right to theft. Recognition of a right to health would obligate the state to prevent individuals from depriving each other of their health, just as recognition of the two other rights now prevents them from depriving others of their liberty and property. It would also obligate the state to respect the health of the individual and to deprive him of this asset only in accordance with due process of law, just as it now respects the individual's liberty and property and deprives him of them only in accordance with due process of law.

As matters now stand, the state not only fails to protect the individual's health, but it actually hinders him in his efforts to safeguard his own health; for example, it permits both industries and individuals to befoul the air we breathe. Furthermore, the state also prohibits individuals from obtaining medical care from certain officially unqualified experts and from buying and ingesting certain officially dangerous drugs. Sometimes, the state deliberately deprives the individual of treatment under the very guise of providing treatment.[20]

To be sure, there are good reasons, in an age in which the powerful centralized state is idolized as the source of all benefits, why the concept of a right to treatment is regarded as progressive and is popular and why the concept of a right to health has, so far as I know, never even been articulated, much less recognized by legislators and courts. On the one hand, recognition of a right to health rather than to treatment would impose greater obligations on the state to insure domestic peace, especially the protection from theft of an individual's health as a type of private property; on the other hand, it would impose greater restraints on its own powers vis-à-vis the citizen, especially on its jurisdiction over the licensure of physicians and the dispensing of drugs. Such a government would have to shoulder greater responsibilities for its duties as policeman, while it would have to limit its alleged responsibilities for dispensing services—in short, the very antithesis of the type of state that modern liberal social reformers consider desirable and necessary for the attainment of their goals. Instead of fostering the independent judgment of the individual, such reformers encourage his submission to an ostensibly competent and benevolent authority; hence, they project the image of medical therapist onto the state, while casting the citizen in the complementary role of sick patient. That of course places the individual in precisely that inferior and submissive role vis-à-vis the government from which the founding fathers sought, by means of the Constitution, to rescue him. Politically, the right to treatment is thus simply the right to submit to authority—a right that has always been dear both to those in power and those incapable of managing their own lives.

20. See, for example, "Testing Synanon," *Time*, July 12, 1968, p. 74.

The state can protect and promote the interests of its sick, or potentially sick, citizens in one of two ways: either by coercing physicians, and other medical and paramedical personnel, to serve patients—as state-owned slaves, in the last analysis; or by creating economic, moral, and political circumstances favorable to a plentiful suply of competent physicians and effective drugs—letting individuals care for their bodies as they care for their other possessions.

The former solution corresponds to and reflects efforts to solve human problems by recourse to the all-powerful state. The rights promised by such a state—exemplified by the right to treatment—are not opportunities for uncoerced choices by individuals, but powers vested in the state for the subjection of the interests of one group to those of another.[21]

The latter solution corresponds to and reflects efforts to solve human problems by recourse to individual initiative and voluntary association without interference by the state. The rights exacted from such a state—exemplified by the right to life, liberty, and health—are limitations on its own powers and sphere of action and provide the conditions necessary for, but of course do not insure the proper exercise of, free and responsible individual choices.

In these two solutions, we recognize the fundamental polarities of the great ideological conflict of our age, perhaps of all ages, and of the human condition itself—individualism and capitalism on the one side, collectivism and communism on the other. *Tertium non datur*. There is no other choice.

21. The position of the physician in Czechoslovakia is illustrative. "The constitution [of Czechoslovakia] declares that health care is a right of the people and that it is the duty of the state to satisfy that right." In practice, that right is assured through "the assignment [by the state] of a low economic (productive) status to the health services. . . . A skilled factory worker may earn much more than a doctor through premium pay. Even a taxi driver may earn more than a doctor. . . . Almost universal was the comment: 'We are not attracting the best people into medicine' " (J. D. Cooper, "Czechoslovakia Reflects Regional Plan Problems," *Hospital Tribune*, September 9, 1968, pp. 1, 16).

# 9

# Justice in the Therapeutic State

The concept of justice and the concept of treatment belong to two different frames of references or realms of discourse—the former to law and morals, the latter to medicine and health. Both justice and treatment articulate ideas basic to human life; both have dual uses—one popular, the other technical. Although justice is closely linked with, and receives its most precise meaning from, the workings of the legal system, the concept is not the private property of lawyers but belongs to everyone. Similarly, although treatment is closely linked with, and receives its most precise meaning from, the workings of the medical profession, the concept is not the private property of physicians but belongs to everyone. I shall be concerned here with examining the relations between these two concepts in an effort to clarify currently popular and prevalent attempts to assimilate jurisprudence to science, law to medicine, the judge to the physician, and justice to treatment.

Law and medicine are among the oldest and most revered professions. That is because each articulates and promotes a basic human need and value—social cooperation in the case of law, health in that of medicine. Simply put, the law opposes some types of social processes: it calls them *crimes* and imposes punishment on those who commit them. Likewise, medicine combats some types of bodily processes: it calls them *diseases* and offers treatment to those who suffer from them.

To exist as a person is synonymous with existing as a social being. The regulation of social relations is an indispensable feature of every society and indeed of every coming together of two or more individuals. The concept of justice is thus necessary both for the regulation of human relations and for judging the moral quality of the resulting situation. That is what is meant by the statement that without law there can be no justice but that the law itself may be unjust.

What constitutes justice varies from place to place and from time to time. The variance does not prove that the concept is devoid of meaning or is unscientific—as some contemporary social scientists claim. Instead, it shows that to the question, What is a good or proper social order? mankind has given, and continues to give, not one but many answers. For example, in principle at least, capitalists believe that those who work harder or produce more, or whose services are more valuable to the community, should receive more for their work than those whose efforts are less productive; whereas Communists believe that the products of all individuals should be pooled and distributed on the basis of the Marxist formula "From each according to his abilities, to each according to his needs."

Framed as general rules of the game of life, contrasting concepts of justice such as those listed above would seem to have nothing in common. That is a fallacy. For what underlies all concepts of justice is a notion so basic to social intercourse that without it life would promptly degenerate into a Hobbesian war of all against all. The notion common to all diverse concepts of justice is *reciprocity*—that is, the expectation that we shall keep our promises to others and they shall keep theirs to us. "It is confessedly unjust," wrote John Stuart Mill, "to *break faith* with any one: to violate an engagement, either express or implied, or to disappoint expectations raised by our own conduct."[1] More recently, Paul Freund has similarly sought to locate the core of justice in the concept of contract. He writes that "the concept of contract is a paradigm case of justice viewed as the satisfaction of reasonable expectations."[2]

1. J. S. Mill, *Utilitarianism*, in *Essential Works of John Stuart Mill*, ed. M. Lerner (New York: Bantam Books, 1961), p. 230.
2. P. A. Freund, "Social Justice and the Law," in R. B. Brandt, ed., *Social Justice* (Englewood Cliffs, N.J.: Prentice-Hall, 1962), p. 95.

Why is contract so all-important to human life? Because it is the foremost rational, nonviolent instrument for the equalization of social power. Contract is the social device *par excellence* that liberates the relatively powerless individual (or group) from domination by his more powerful superiors, thus freeing him to plan for the future. Conversely, lack of contract, or systematic contract violation, is an essential characteristic of oppression: deprived of the power to plan for the future, the inferior individual (or group) becomes subjected to the status derogation of dependency by his superiors. Thus, when the future arrives, the oppressed individual will be unable to care for himself and will be dependent on his protectors (for example, parents, politicians, psychiatrists).

To be sure, like all social arrangements, contract favors some members of the group and frustrates others. Specifically, it favors the weak (that is, those who lack the power to coerce or, if they possess such power, the will to use it), and it frustrates the strong (that is, those who have such power or, if they lack it, strive to possess it). Generally, then, contract favors the child as against the parent, the employee as against the employer, and the individual as against the state. In each of those relationships (and in other similar situations), the superior member of the pair does not require contract to plan for his future: he can control his partner, by brute force if necessary. In short, contract expands the self-determination of the weak by constricting the powers of the strong to coerce him; at the same time, by placing the value of abiding by the terms of a contract above that of naked power and by universalizing that value, contract tames not only the power of the strong to coerce but also that of the weak to countercoerce.

In political life, the paradigm of contract is the rule of law, the principle that limits interferences by the state in the conduct of the individual to circumstances that are clearly defined and known in advance to the individual. By avoiding law breaking, the citizen can thus feel secure from unexpected interference by state power. That arrangement may be contrasted with despotic or tyrannical government, whose principal characteristic in its dealings with the individual is not harshness but rather arbitrariness. Indeed, the brutality and terror of that kind of political arrangement lie precisely in the utter unpredictability with which the police power of the state may be deployed against the individual.

One more example of the fundamental role of contract in the concept of justice should suffice. It is an ancient legal maxim that there should be no punishment without law (*Nulla poena sine lege*). The principle that a person should not be punished for an act that was not prohibited by law at the time when he engaged in it shows dramatically that the concept of justice is rooted in ideas and sentiments that have more to do with the need to make behavior predictable than with the need to protect society from harm. For, clearly, a person may harm his neighbor without his behavior's qualifying as an act prohibited by law. Arguing from the allegedly scientific point of view, the modern psychiatrist or behavioral scientist would hold that what is—or ought to be—important here is the proper restraint and remotivation of the malefactor, not the abstract idea of justice. Hence, he needs no preexisting law to justify invoking the social sanction he calls psychiatric treatment. Indeed, it is precisely at this point that the behavioral scientist falls back on the analogy between misbehavior and illness by arguing that just as a person may fall ill without his condition being officially recognized by medical science in the form of a diagnosis, so too he may engage in "dangerous" conduct without his behavior being officially recognized by the law as a criminal act. In that view, what determines the existence of the undesired condition, whether it be disease or deviance, illness or crime—and what justifies social intervention against it, whether it be treatment or punishment, medical hospitalization or mental hospitalization—is the judgment of the expert, not a rule written down by lawmakers and legitimized by the judicial and political processes of government.

These two fundamental principles of regulating human relations—the contractual and the discretionary—serve different aims. Each acquires its value from its function—to foster the individual's capacity for independence by enabling him to plan for the future in the case of contract, and to enable the expert to act with optimal effectiveness by freeing him from the limitations of restricting rules in the case of discretion. Since those are two radically different ends, it is hardly surprising that each requires different means for its attainment.

Man is not only a person, a social being; he is also an animal, a biological organism. Hence, his biological equipment—that is, his body—which is a necessary but not a sufficient condition for his role as a person, will also be of paramount importance to him. For if a person's body is injured or becomes diseased, his ability to perform his social and personal functions will be altered, impaired, or even destroyed; and if his body ceases to function altogether, then he ceases to exist as a member of the group or as a person. Thus, just as the law has come into being to regulate and safeguard man's relations to his fellow man, so medicine has come into being to regulate and safeguard his relation to his own body.

Inasmuch as these two basic human needs are closely related—man's relations to his body always occurring in a context of preexisting social regulations—it is not surprising that law and medicine (their concepts, interventions, and sometimes their personnel) are often intertwined and that during various historical periods each of these disciplines has made deep inroads into the territory of the other. In the Middle Ages, for example, when the religious ideology ruled undisputed over the minds of men, the scope and function of the medical healer was strictly circumscribed by the authority of the Church. Not only the dissection of bodies, but also the use of drugs was thus forbidden as contrary to the will of God. Hence it was that medicine, independent of the teachings and powers of the Church, was in the hands of Arab and Jewish physicians or was practiced illegally by white witches. Similarly, in our day, when a medical-psychiatric ideology rules undisputed over the minds of men, legal concepts and methods of social control are confused with, and corrupted by, medical concepts and methods of social control. The upshot is the transformation of the state from a legal and political entity into a medical and therapeutic one.[3]

3. In this connection, see my *The Manufacture of Madness: A Comparative Study of the Inquisition and the Mental Health Movement* (New York: Harper & Row, 1970) and *Ideology and Insanity: Essays on the Psychiatric Dehumanization of Man* (Garden City, N.Y.: Doubleday, Anchor Press, 1970).

The impetus that drives men to depoliticize and therapeuticize human relations and social conflicts appears to be the same as that which drives them to comprehend and control the physical world. The history of this process—that is, of the birth of modern science in the seventeenth century and its rise to ideological hegemony in the twentieth—has been adequately set forth by others.[4] I shall confine myself here to illustrating the incipient and developed forms of this ideology through quotations from the works of two of its most illustrious American protagonists—Benjamin Rush and Karl Menninger.

Benjamin Rush (1745–1813) signed the Declaration of Independence, was physician general of the Continental Army, and served as professor of physic and dean of the medical school at the University of Pennsylvania. He is the undisputed father of American psychiatry: his portrait adorns the official seal of the American Psychiatric Association. I shall list without comment passages from Rush's writings that show how he transformed moral questions into medical problems and political judgments into therapeutic decisions.

> Perhaps hereafter it may be as much the business of a physician as it is now of a divine to reclaim mankind from vice.[5]

> Mankind considered as creatures made for immortality are worthy of all our cares. Let us view them as patients in a hospital. The more they resist our efforts to serve them, the more they have need of our services.[6]

> Miss H. L. . . . was confined in our hospital in the year 1800. For several weeks she discovered [displayed] every mark of a sound mind, except one. She hated her father. On a certain day, she acknowledged,

4. For example, see F. A. Hayek, *The Counter-Revolution of Science: Studies on the Abuse of Reason* (New York: Free Press, 1964), and F. Matson, *The Broken Image: Man, Science, and Society* (New York: Braziller, 1964).

5. Benjamin Rush to Granville Sharp, July 9, 1774, in J. A. Woods, ed., "The Correspondence of Benjamin Rush and Granville Sharp, 1773–1809," *Journal of American Studies* 1 (April 1967): 8.

6. Rush to Granville Sharp, November 28, 1783, ibid., p. 20.

with pleasure, a return of her filial attachment and affection for him; soon after she was discharged cured.[7]

Physicians [are the] best judges of sanity. . . .

Suicide is madness. . . .

Chagrin, shame, fear, terror, anger, unfit[ness] for legal acts, are transient madness.[8]

Lying is a corporeal disease. . . . Persons thus diseased cannot speak the truth upon any subject.[9]

Terror acts powerfully upon the body, through the medium of the mind, and should be employed in the cure of madness.[10]

There was a time when these things [criticism of Rush's opinions and actions] irritated and distressed me, but I now hear and see them with the same indifference and pity that I hear the ravings and witness the antic gestures of my deranged patients in our Hospital. We often hear of "prisoners at large." The majority of mankind are *madmen at large*.[11]

Were we to live our lives over again and engage in the same benevolent enterprise [political reform], our means should not be reasoning but bleeding, purging, low diet, and the tranquilizing chair.[12]

Rush's foregoing views provide an early nineteenth-century example of the medical-therapeutic perspective on political and social conduct. His statements amply support my contention that although ostensibly he was a founder of American constitutional government, actually he was an architect of the therapeutic state.[13] The leaders of the American Enlightenment never tired of emphasizing the

7. Rush, *Medical Inquiries and Observations upon the Diseases of the Mind* (1812; New York: Macmillan, Hafner Press, 1962), pp. 255–256.

8. Rush, "Lecture on the Medical Jurisprudence of the Mind" (1810), in *The Autobiography of Benjamin Rush: His "Travels through Life" Together with His "Commonplace Book for 1789–1812"*, ed. G. W. Corner (Princeton, N.J.: Princeton University Press, 1948), p. 350.

9. Rush, *Medical Inquiries*, p. 265.

10. Ibid., p. 175.

11. Rush, *Letters of Benjamin Rush*, ed. L. H. Butterfield (Princeton, N.J.: Princeton University Press, 1951), vol 2, p. 1090.

12. Ibid., p. 1092.

13. See my *Law, Liberty, and Psychiatry: An Inquiry into the Social Uses of Mental Health Practices* (New York: Macmillan, 1963), esp. pp. 212–222.

necessity for restraining the powers of the rulers—that is, for checks and balances in the structure of government. Rush, on the other hand, consistently advocated rule by benevolent despotism—that is, political absolutism justified as medical necessity.

In short, as the Constitution articulates the principles of the legal state, in which both ruler and ruled are governed by the rule of law; so Rush's writings articulate the principles of the therapeutic state, in which the citizen-patient's conduct is governed by the clinical judgment of the medical despot. The former constitutes a basis for expanding the personal liberty of the citizen; the latter, for expanding the political power of the government.

To bring into focus the ideology and rhetoric on which our present-day therapeutic society rests, I shall next present in capsule form the pertinent opinions of one of its foremost contemporary spokesmen, Karl Menninger.

Karl Menninger (b. 1893) is a founder of the famed Menninger Clinic and Foundation, a former president of the American Psychoanalytic Association, the recipient of numerous psychiatric honors, and the author of several influential books in the mental-health field. Like Rush before him, Menninger is one of the most prominent psychiatrists in America. His views illustrate the contemporary psychiatric mode of viewing all manner of human problems as mental illnesses—indeed, all of life as a disease requiring psychiatric care. The following quotations point up that view.

> . . . the declamation continues about travesties upon *justice* that result from the introduction of psychiatric methods into courts. But what science or scientist is interested in *justice?* Is pneumonia just? Or cancer? . . . The scientist is seeking the amelioration of an unhappy situation. This can be secured only if the scientific laws controlling the situation can be discovered and complied with, and not by talking of "justice." . . .[14]

> Prostitution and homosexuality rank high in the kingdom of evils.[15] From the standpoint of the psychiatrist, both homosexuality and

14. K. Menninger, *The Human Mind*, 3rd ed. (New York: Knopf, 1966), p. 449.

15. Menninger, Introduction to *The Wolfenden Report: Report of the Committee on Homosexual Offenses and Prostitution* (New York: Stein & Day, 1964), p. 5.

prostitution—and add to this the use of prostitutes—constitute evidence of immature sexuality and either arrested psychological development or regression. Whatever it may be called by the public, there is no question in the minds of psychiatrists regarding the abnormality of such behavior.[16]

. . . in the unconscious mind, it [masturbation] always represents an aggression against someone.[17]

Eliminating one offender who happens to get caught *weakens* public security by creating a false sense of diminished danger through a definite remedial measure. Actually, it does not remedy anything, and it bypasses completely the real and unsolved problem of how to identify, detect, and detain potentially dangerous citizens.[18]

The principle of *no* punishment cannot allow of any exception; it must apply in every case, even the worst case, the most horrible case, the most dreadful case—not merely in the accidental, sympathy-arousing case.[19]

When the community begins to look upon the expression of aggressive violence as the symptom of an illness or as indicative of illness, it will be because it believes doctors can do something to correct such a condition. At present, some better-informed individuals do believe and expect this.[20]

Do I believe there is effective treatment for offenders . . . ? Most certainly and definitely I do. Not all cases, to be sure. . . . Some provision has to be made for incurables—pending new knowledge—and these will include some offenders. But I believe the majority of them would prove to be curable. The willfulness and the viciousness of offenders are part of the thing for which they have to be treated. They must not thwart our therapeutic attitude. It is simply not true that most of them are "fully aware" of what they are doing, nor is it true that they want no help from anyone, although some of them say so.[21]

16. Ibid., p. 6.
17. Menninger, *Man against Himself* (New York: Harcourt Brace Jovanovich, 1938), p. 61.
18. Menninger, *The Crime of Punishment* (New York: Viking Press, 1968), p. 108.
19. Ibid., p. 207.
20. Ibid., p. 257.
21. Ibid., pp. 260–261.

> Some mental patients must be detained for a time even against their wishes, and the same is true of offenders.[22]

As the foregoing quotations show, Menninger focuses systematically on the offender, or alleged offender, who, in his view, is either punished with hostile intention or treated with therapeutic intention. Accordingly, he urges that we abandon the legal and penological system with its limited and prescribed penalties and substitute for it a medical and therapeutic system with unlimited and discretionary sanctions defined as treatments.

In short, the enlightened behavioral technologist has for centuries sought the destruction of law and justice and their replacement by science and therapy.

Those who see the main domestic business of the state as the maintenance of internal peace through a system of just laws justly administered and those who see it as the provision of behavioral reform scientifically administered by a scientific elite have, in fact, two radically different visions of society and of man. Since each of these groups strives after a different goal, it is not surprising that each condemns the other's methods; constitutional government, the rule of law, and due process are indeed inefficient means for inspiring the personality change of criminals, especially if their crime is not shoplifting (which is Menninger's favorite example), but violating laws regulating contraception, abortion, drug abuse, or homosexuality. Similarly, unlimited psychiatric discretion over the identification and diagnosis of alleged offenders, coercive therapeutic interventions, and lifelong incarceration in an insane asylum are neither effective nor ethical means for protecting individual liberties or insuring restraints on the powers of the government, especially when the individual's "illness" is despair over his inconsequential life and the wish to put an end to it.

The legal and the medical approaches to social control represent two radically different ideologies, each with its own justificatory rhetoric and restraining actions. It behooves us to understand clearly the differences between them.

In the legal concept of the state, justice is both an end and a means; when such a state is just, it may be said to have fulfilled its

22. Ibid., p. 265.

domestic function. It has then no further claims on its citizens (save for defense against external aggression). What people do—whether they are virtuous or wicked, healthy or sick, rich or poor, educated or stupid—is none of the state's business. This, then, is a concept of the state as an institution of limited scope and powers. (In such a state, the people are, of course, not restrained from fulfilling their needs not met by the state through voluntary associations.)

In the scientific-technological concept of the state, therapy is only a means, not an end: the goal of the therapeutic state is universal health, or at least unfailing relief from suffering. The untroubled condition of man and society is a quintessential feature of the medical-therapeutic perspective on politics: conflict among individuals, and especially between the individual and the state, is invariably seen as a symptom of illness or psychopathology; and the primary function of the state is accordingly the removal of such conflict through appropriate therapy—imposed by force if necessary. It is not difficult to recognize in the imagery of the therapeutic state the old inquisitional, or the more recent totalitarian, concept of the state, now clothed in the garb of psychiatric treatment.

Whether we want a society in which man has a chance, however small, to develop his powers and to become an individual or one in which such individualism is considered to be evil and man (if we may call him that) is fashioned into a plastic, compliant robot by his scientific masters is, in the last analysis, a basic ethical question to which we cannot, and need not, address ourselves here. Of course, all who feel deeply about either of these alternatives believe that they are championing man's dearest and most authentic aspirations. According to the libertarians, more than anything else man needs protection from the dangers of unlimited government; according to the therapeutists, he needs protection from the dangers of unlimited illness. Moreover, as so often happens when people become separated by an ideological gulf, the advocates of these two points of view are no longer on speaking terms. In particular, the behavioral engineers and psychiatric therapists, who have succeeded in defining their position as the progressive and scientific one, have ceased even to acknowledge the existence of a large body of fact and thought critical of what I call the "theory and practice of psychiatric violence." That was true of Rush nearly two hundred years ago, who in his writings never engaged those who opposed tyranny, whether priestly or medical; and it is true now of Menninger, who never confronts those who fear and distrust the violence of psychiatrists no less than of politicians.

Among contemporary scholars and thinkers who have opposed the behavioristic-scientistic forces tending toward the "abolition of man," C. S. Lewis stands very high indeed. Until his death in 1963, Lewis was professor of medieval and Renaissance English at Cambridge University. He is probably best known for his book *The Screwtape Letters*, which first established him as an influential spokesman for Christianity in the English-speaking world and a brilliant critic of modern science and technology as dehumanizing social institutions.[23] I list below passages illustrative of Lewis's views pertinent to the relations between psychiatry and law.

> I am not supposing them [the Conditioners] to be bad men. They are, rather, not men (in the old sense) at all. They are, if you like, men who have sacrificed their own share in traditional humanity in order to devote themselves to the task of deciding what "Humanity" shall henceforth mean. . . . Nor are their subjects necessarily unhappy men. They are not men at all: they are artefacts. Man's final conquest has proved to be the abolition of Man.[24]

> . . . when we cease to consider what the criminal deserves and consider only what will cure him or deter others, we have tacitly removed him from the sphere of justice altogether; instead of a person, a subject of rights, we now have a mere object, a patient, a "case."[25]

> The first result of the Humanitarian theory is, therefore, to substitute for a definite sentence (reflecting to some extent the community's moral judgment on the degree of ill-desert involved) an indefinite sentence terminable only by the word of those experts . . . who inflict it. Which of us, if he stood in the dock, would not prefer to be tried by the old system?[26]

23. C. S. Lewis, *The Screwtape Letters and Screwtape Proposes a Toast* (New York: Macmillan, 1967).

24. Lewis, *The Abolition of Man* (New York: Macmillan, 1965), pp. 76–77.

25. Lewis, "The Humanitarian Theory of Punishment," *Res Judicatae* (Melbourne University, Melbourne, Australia), vol. 6 (1953): 225.

26. Ibid., p. 226

> Of all tyrannies a tyranny sincerely exercised for the good of its victims may be the most oppressive. . . . To be "cured" against one's will and cured of states which we may not regard as disease is to be put on a level with those who have not yet reached the age of reason or those who never will; to be classed with infants, imbeciles, and domestic animals. But to be punished, however severely, because we have deserved it, because we "ought to have known better," is to be treated as a human person made in God's image.[27]

> For if crime and disease are to be regarded as the same thing, it follows that any state of mind which our masters choose to call "disease" can be treated as a crime; and compulsorily cured. . . . but under the Humanitarian theory it will not be called by the shocking name of Persecution. . . . The new Nero will approach us with the silky manners of a doctor. . . . Even if the treatment is painful, even if it is life-long, even if it is fatal, that will be only a regretable accident; the intention was purely therapeutic.[28]

But the Humanitarians remain undaunted. Fifteen years after Lewis wrote the passages just quoted, Menninger declares: "The secret of success in all [penological] programs, however, is the replacement of the punitive attitude with the therapeutic attitude. A therapeutic attitude is essential regardless of the particular form of treatment or help."[29]

The decision whether to treat others justly (fairly) or therapeutically (benevolently) is not a choice facing only jurists and psychiatrists; on the contrary, it is a choice everyone must make. The way an individual responds to that challenge, the choice he makes, largely shapes and defines his moral character. Some choose justice; they are regarded as competent and reliable by their friends and as unyielding by their enemies. Others choose benevolence; they are regarded as kindly and loving by their friends and as despotic by their enemies. That is not to say that individuals cannot, in principle, be both just and benevolent. As persons they may be

27. Ibid., p. 228.
28. Ibid., p. 229.
29. Menninger, *The Crime of Punishment*, p. 262.

both; but when faced with concrete situations, they must often choose between those two values and types of conduct.

The same considerations hold for societies. William Frankena puts it well when he asserts that "societies can be loving, efficient, prosperous, or good, as well as just, but they may well be just without being notably benevolent, efficient, prosperous, or good."[30] He also notes, correctly, that there is an internal contradiction between a state being both loving and just: the more loving it is, the more unjust it must become, and vice versa (unless justice is itself considered a form of love). A "just society," Frankena continues, restating the traditional definition, "is, strictly speaking, not simply a loving one. It must in its actions and institutions fulfill certain formal requirements dictated by reason rather than love: it must be rule-governed."[31] That puts the case of the just state versus the therapeutic state squarely before us. And it helps us see what I consider the fatal flaw—both empirically and ethically—in the argument for love over justice.

As we saw earlier, justice may, in its most basic sense, be readily defined as the fulfillment of contracts or expectations. Contracts, moreover, consist of performances and counterperformances—that is, of overt acts. They thus differ from intentions, sentiments, or states of mind—which are private experiences. Accordingly, justice is open to public inspection, scrutiny, and judgment, whereas love is closed to such examination and evaluation. Hence, the claim that one is acting justly is a plea for the support of the good opinion of others, whereas the claim that one is acting lovingly leaves no room for the judgment of others and in its zeal brooks no opposition. In short, although love appeals to the ideal of consideration for the *needs of others* and justice appeals to the ideal of consideration for *agreed-upon rules*, in actual practice just actions afford more protection for the self-defined interests of others than do loving actions.

I have tried to show that justice and freedom are closely related

30. W. F. Frankena, "The Concept of Social Justice," in Brandt, ed., *Social Justice*, p. 3.
31. Ibid., p. 23.

concepts and that the value of the former is contingent on that of the latter. Thus, if freedom is debased, so is justice.

I use the term *freedom* to signify man's ability to make uncoerced choices. In that sense of the term, freedom is endangered from two different directions, by two different kinds of threats. One threat emanates from within the individual, from the limitations of his body, his mind, and his personality; for example, illness and stupidity diminish or impair freedom by diminishing or impairing man's capacity to formulate or execute uncoerced choices. Another threat emanates from outside the individual, from the limitations of his worldly, and especially his social, circumstances; for example, other men, acting either as individuals or through the coercive apparatus of the church or the state, diminish or impair freedom by diminishing or impairing man's capacity to formulate or execute uncoerced choices.

To confuse these two sources of danger to individual liberties is fatal to their cause. Yet that is precisely what the modern liberal and scientific social critic and reformer often does: by stressing the similarities rather than the differences between man's vulnerability at the hands of nature and of the state, between the injury inflicted on a person by an illness and by an individual, the behavioral scientist technicizes human problems and thus transforms man into a thing. Having done that at the outset, what is there left for him to protect? Nothing but an image, a shadow—which he then casts into the role of the alleged beneficiary of his spiritual munificence. In that way, the behavioral technologist authenticates himself as a great healer and a great scientist. But his performance is a tragic farce, a playact not unlike that of the child or so-called madman: in each of these cases, the performer impersonates an important or noble actor—whether it be fireman, Savior, or physician—and plays his part without regard to the participation of other actors or audience. It is this lack of confirmation by their respective beneficiaries—of child as fireman, of madman as Jesus, and of humanitarian institutional psychiatrist as healer—that defines each of these roles as counterfeit. But there is this difference for the psychiatrist: whereas child and madman lack the power to impose their role playing on unconsenting others (thus usually having to confine their performances to their families), psychiatrists, invested with the coercive powers of the state, often impose their definitions of reality on others.[32] Hence, in the therapeutic state, care, help, and treatment are not what the involuntary patients request, but what the humanitarian psychiatrists impose.

What, then, of justice in the therapeutic state? Its fate may be varied, but of this we can be certain: it will cease to exist as we have come to know it. Justice may thus be consigned to the history books as the relic of a barbarous age that valued individual freedom more highly than collective security, or it may be redefined in the newspeak of our times as treatment.

32. See generally my *The Myth of Mental Illness: Foundations of a Theory of Personal Conduct*, rev. ed. (New York: Harper & Row, 1974), esp. pp. 241–249.

# 10

# The Illogic and Immorality of Involuntary Psychiatric Interventions: A Personal Restatement

Involuntary mental hospitalization—or compulsory admission to hospital, as it is called in England—is the paradigmatic policy of psychiatry. Whenever and wherever psychiatry has been recognized and practiced as the medical specialty dealing with the treatment of insanity, madness, or mental disease, then and there persons have been incarcerated in insane asylums, madhouses, or mental hospitals.[1]

In recent years, this deprivation of liberty has been justified on two different grounds, one more popular in America, the other in England. In the United States, the defenders of involuntary psychiatry claim that mental health is more important than personal freedom and that the well-being of the individual and the nation justify certain psychiatric infringements on individual liberty. In England, its defenders, sidestepping the dilemma of such a rank-ordering of values, claim that the civil-liberties problem inherent in compulsory mental hospitalization is now so small as to be insignificant.[2]

In the American view, then, compulsory psychiatric confinement

1. See my (ed.) *The Age of Madness: The History of Involuntary Mental Hospitalization Presented in Selected Texts* (Garden City, N.Y.: Doubleday, Anchor Press, 1973).

2. See my "The ACLU's 'Mental Illness' Cop-Out," *Reason* 5 (January 1974): 4–9, and Preface to the British Edition, *The Age of Madness* (London: Routledge & Kegan Paul, 1975), pp. xv–xviii.

is a sort of limited martial law; while in the British view, it is a sort of dead-letter law. But mental patients do not menace society so gravely as to justify suppressing them by extralegal measures, nor are they suppressed so rarely as to justify our regarding the measures used against them as moribund.

Because involuntary mental hospitalization continues to be the paradigmatic practice of coercive or institutional psychiatry, it seems to me worthwhile to recapitulate briefly the justifications for its legitimacy advanced by its supporters and the justifications for its illegitimacy that I have advanced.

The coercion and restraint of the mental patient by the psychiatrist—or, better, of the madman by the alienist, as these protagonists were first called—is coeval with the origin and development of psychiatry. As a discrete discipline, psychiatry began in the seventeenth century with the building of insane asylums, first in France, then throughout the civilized world. These institutions were of course prisons in which were confined not only so-called madmen but all of society's undesirables—abandoned children, prostitutes, incurably sick persons, the aged and indigent.[3]

How did people in general, and those directly responsible for these confinements—the legislators and jurists, the physicians and the victims' relatives—in particular justify such incarceration of persons not guilty of criminal offenses? The answer is: by means of the imagery and rhetoric of madness, insanity, psychosis, schizophrenia, mental illness—call it what you will—which transformed the inmate into a patient, his prison into a hospital, and his warden into a doctor. Characteristically, the first official proposition of the Association of Medical Superintendents of American Institutions for the Insane, the organization that became in 1921 the American Psychiatric Association, was, "Resolved, that it is the unanimous sense of this convention that the attempt to abandon entirely the use of all means of personal restraint is not sanctioned by the true interests of the insane."[4]

3. See my *The Manufacture of Madness: A Comparative Study of the Inquisition and the Mental Health Movement* (New York: Harper & Row, 1970), pp. 13–16.

4. Quoted in N. Ridenour, *Mental Health in the United States: A Fifty-Year History* (Cambridge, Mass.: Harvard University Press, 1961), p. 76.

Ever since then, this paternalistic justification of psychiatric coercion has been a prominent theme in psychiatry, not only in America but throughout the world. Thus, in 1967—123 years after the drafting of its first resolution—the American Psychiatric Association reaffirmed its support of psychiatric coercion and restraint. In its "Position Statement on the Question of the Adequacy of Treatment," the association declared that "restraints may be imposed [on the patient] from within by pharmacologic means or by locking the door of a ward. Either imposition may be a legitimate component of a treatment program."[5]

The British Mental Health Act of 1959 provides medico-legal measures for both civil and criminal commitment virtually identical to those of the various American states. Part IV of the act, entitled "Compulsory Admission to Hospital and Guardianship," articulates the criteria for civil commitment as follows: "An application for admission for observation may be made in respect of a patient on the grounds (*a*) that he is suffering from mental disorder of a nature or degree which warrants the detention of the patient in a hospital under observation . . . (*b*) that he ought to be so detained in the interests of his own health or safety or with a view to the protection of other persons."[6]

Justifications for involuntary psychiatric interventions of all kinds—and especially for involuntary mental hospitalization—similar to those accepted in the United States and the United Kingdom are, of course, advanced in other countries. In short, just as involuntary servitude had been accepted for millennia as a proper economic and social arrangement, so involuntary psychiatry has been accepted for centuries as a proper medical and therapeutic arrangement.

It is this entire system of interlocking psychiatric ideas and insituations, justifications and practices, that for some twenty years I have analyzed and attacked. I have described and documented the precise legal status of the mental-hospital patient—as an innocent

5. Council of the American Psychiatric Association, "Position Statement on the Question of the Adequacy of Treatment," *American Journal of Psychiatry* 123 (May 1967): 1459.

6. *Mental Health Act, 1959*, 7 and 8 Eliz. 2, Ch. 72 (London: Her Majesty's Stationery Office, 1959), p. 15.

person incarcerated in a psychiatric prison; articulated my objections to institutional psychiatry—as an extralegal system of penology and punishments; and demonstrated what seems to me, in a free society, our only morally proper option with respect to the problem of so-called psychiatric abuses—namely, the complete abolition of all involuntary psychiatric interventions.

My objections to the principles and practices upon which involuntary psychiatric interventions rest may be summarized as follows:

The term *mental illness* is a metaphor. More particularly, as this term is used in mental-hygiene legislation, *mental illness* is not the name of a medical disease or disorder but is a quasi-medical label whose purpose is to conceal conflict as illness and to justify coercion as treatment.

If mental illness is a bona fide illness—"like any other," as official medical, psychiatric, and mental-health organizations such as the World Health Organization, the American and British medical associations, and the American Psychiatric Association maintain—then it follows, logically and linguistically, that it must be treated like any other illness. Hence, mental-hygiene laws must be repealed. There are no special laws for patients with peptic ulcer or pneumonia; why then should there be special laws for patients with depression or schizophrenia?

If, on the other hand, mental illness is, as I contend, a metaphor and a myth, then it also follows that mental-hygiene laws should be repealed.

Further, if there were no mental-hygiene laws—which create a category of individuals who, though officially labeled as mentally ill, would prefer not to be subjected to involuntary psychiatric interventions—then the misdeeds now committed by those who care for mental patients could not arise or endure.

In short, all those who draft and administer laws pertaining to involuntary psychiatric interventions should be regarded as the adversaries, not the allies, of the so-called mental patient. Civil libertarians, and indeed all men and women who believe that no one may be justly deprived of liberty except upon conviction for a crime, should oppose all forms of involuntary psychiatric interventions.

What, then, are some of the most important objections to my contention that mental disorders are not bona fide diseases and to my claim that imprisonment for insanity, as opposed to lawbreaking, is incompatible with the moral principles of a free society?

First, some of my critics say that I am wrong because what we now call mental diseases may yet be shown to be caused, at least in some cases, by subtle pathophysiological processes in the body—in particular, by disorders in the molecular chemistry of the brain—that we do not yet know how to measure or record. Nevertheless, such processes, like those responsible for the psychoses associated with paresis or pellagra, exist (so runs this argument), and it is only because of the present state of our knowledge, or rather ignorance, that we cannot yet properly diagnose them. But such an advance in the science and technology of medical diagnosis would only add to the list of literal diseases and would not in the slightest impair the validity of my argument that when we call certain kinds of disapproved behaviors mental diseases, we create a category of metaphorical diseases. This type of objection to my views, which actually represents just another instance of biological reductionism, misses the point I try to make; to uphold it would be like upholding the view that because certain canvases thought to be forged Renoirs or Cézannes prove to be, on closer study, genuine, all forged masterpieces are genuine. If there are real or literal diseases, there must also be others that are fake or metaphorical.

Second, other critics say that I am wrong, not because I say that mental illnesses are unlike bodily illnesses (an assertion with which they claim to agree), nor because I say that involuntary hospitalization or treatment is no more justified for so-called mental illness than it is for bodily illness (a moral principle with which they also claim to be in sympathy), but because the term *mental illness* often designates a phenomenologically identifiable and hence valid category of conduct. But I do not deny that. I have never maintained that the conduct of a depressed or elated person is the same as that of a person who is contented and even-tempered or that the conduct of a person who claims to be Jesus or Napoleon is the same as that of one who makes no such false claims. I object to psychiatric diagnostic terms not because they are meaningless, but because they are used to stigmatize, dehumanize, imprison, and torture those to whom they are applied. To put it somewhat differently, I oppose involuntary psychiatry, or the rape of the patient by the psychiatrist; but I do not oppose voluntary psychiatry, or psychiatric activities between consenting adults.

The idea that a person accused of crime is innocent until proven guilty is not shared by people everywhere but is, as I need hardly belabor, characteristically English in its historical origin and singularly Anglo-American in its consistent social application. And so is its corollary—that an individual has an inalienable right to personal liberty unless he has been duly convicted in court of an offense punishable by imprisonment. Because this magnificent edifice of dignity and liberty is undermined by psychiatry, I consider the abolition of involuntary psychiatric interventions to be an especially important link in the chain I have tried to forge for restraining this mortal enemy of individualism and self-determination. I hope that my work will help people to discriminate between two types of physicians: those who heal, not so much because they are saints but because *that is their job*; and those who harm, not so much because they are sinners but because *that is their job*. And if some doctors harm—torture rather than treat, murder the soul rather than minister to the body—that is, in part, because society, through the state, asks them, and pays them, to do so.

We saw it happen in Nazi Germany, and we hanged many of the doctors. We see it happen in the Soviet Union, and we denounce the doctors with righteous indignation. But when will we see that the same things are happening in the so-called free societies? When will we recognize—and publicly identify—the medical criminals among us? Or is the very possibility of perceiving many of our leading psychiatrists and psychiatric institutions in that way precluded by the fact that they represent the officially correct views and practices; by the fact that they have the ears of our lawyers and legislators, journalists and judges; and by the fact that they control the vast funds, collected by the state through taxing citizens, that finance an enterprise whose basic moral legitimacy I have called into question?

# 11

# The Metaphors of Faith and Folly

In the Middle Ages, the lives and languages of people were suffused with the imagery of God and permeated by the ideology of Christianity; today, they are suffused with the imagery of science and permeated by the ideology of medicine. That is why the metaphors of the family formerly played an extremely important role in the practical affairs of men and women and why the metaphors of illness play a similar role in them now.

It seems to me reasonable to assume that a medieval person need not have been a theologian to understand—had he wanted to and had he had the courage to—that the vocabulary of the family was used on him and by him in two quite different senses. It was one thing for him to call his parents *father* and *mother* and his siblings *brother* and *sister*. It was quite another for him to call God his *Father in Heaven* and his parish priest simply *Father*.

Had our hypothetical medieval demetaphorizer wanted to pursue a purely linguistic analysis of religion and religious institutions, he could have quickly discovered that although the Church was said to be God's family, it was not exactly like his own family or any other family that he actually knew. For example, in the families he knew, there were, besides the parents and children, also uncles and aunts, cousins and second cousins, and so forth. But there were no cousins and nephews in the Family. Similarly, God was said to have a Son. Did He also have a liver or kidney? There is no need to go on. That way lay blasphemy then and lies humor now, unless one goes too far and offends.

All I am trying to do in these preliminary remarks is to show that it might have been possible for an ordinary person in a theocratic society to understand the metaphors of faith—that is, to grasp the real character of words borrowed and metaphorized from the family, and to use that supposition as my basis for suggesting that it may be similarly possible for an ordinary person in our therapeutic society to understand the metaphors of folly—that is, to grasp the real character of words borrowed and metaphorized from medicine.

Let us start by considering some aspects of the language of medicine.

The terms *ill* and *sick* are often used interchangeably. For example, we can say, "Jones has pneumonia, he is quite ill." And we can say just as well, "Jones has pneumonia, he is quite sick."

*Ill*, however, has a history and a scope that have nothing to do with medicine or disease. It then means, roughly, *bad*, *unfortunate*, *tragic*, or something of that sort. For example, we can speak of *ill will* or *ill fate*, but we cannot speak of *sick will* or *sick fate*. Moreover, we can speak of *ill health* but cannot substitute *sick* as an adjective for *health*.

On the other hand, *ill* has often a much more restricted implication than *sick*, so that there are many instances in which we can use the latter but not the former term. For example, we don't say, "The tiger is ill," or "The tree is ill," but we do say, "The tiger is sick," or "The tree is sick." Revealingly, the strict use of *ill* is restricted to persons; not even body parts or organs may be ill, although they may be sick. We don't say, "His hand is ill," or "He has an ill hand," but we say, "His hand is sick," or "He has a sick hand."

If we want to convey the idea of *ill* about an animal, a part of the human body, or even an abstract noun, then we use *sick*. Thus, we can say about a person that "his liver is sick," and we can also say that a cat or a car, a television set or a joke, or even a whole society is sick. None of them can be ill, however.

It seems that the only nouns to which we cannot attribute the characteristic or condition of being sick are those which refer to concrete nonliving things that do not affect us. For example, we do not usually say that "the mountain is sick," but we might say that if we were Alpinists threatened by avalanches or rock slides. The sky affects us more often, and hence it is less unusual to say that "the sky looks sick." And if we play table tennis, the equipment always affects us, and it is therefore quite natural to say that "this ping-pong ball is sick." In none of these uses, however, can *ill* replace *sick*.

Qualifying *ill* and *sick* with *mentally* introduces new wrinkles into how those terms can be used and what they mean. Clearly, from a purely linguistic viewpoint, if *mentally ill* meant exactly the same thing as *ill* (as some psychiatric propagandists would have us believe), then the term would not have come into being and could not have retained currency. But that alone need not detain us. What should interest us instead is that *mentally ill* and *mentally sick* tend to function linguistically very much as the metaphorically *sick* functions and not at all as does the literally *sick* or *ill*. (By *metaphorically sick*, I mean that the person uses it to express disapproval or dislike of the referent or attributes some sort of malfunctioning or wrongness to it, whereas by *literally sick* or *ill*, I mean that the person uses it to express the specific idea of some sort of bodily disorder or medical disease.)

The literally or medically *sick* occurs in all tenses and moods and with all sorts of time modifiers; the metaphorically or mentally *sick* does not. For example, we can say all of the following: "Jones is sick; he cannot work." "Jones was sick; he could not work." "Jones has been sick; he has not been working." "Jones had been sick; he missed a lot of work." "Jones will be sick; he will not be at work." "Jones is sick today; he is not working." "Don't get sick, Jones; you don't want to miss work."

When metaphorically *sick* is used explicitly, it has a much more restricted range of tenses. We can say, "The joke is sick," or "The joke was sick." But it would be weird to say, "The joke has been sick," or "The joke will be sick." And it would be absurd to say, "The joke is sick today," or "The joke is often sick."

The psychiatrically or mentally *sick*, which I have long contended is covertly metaphorical, has the same restricted range of use as does the overtly metaphorical *sick*. Thus, we can say, "Jones is mentally sick (or ill); he shot the president," or "Jones was mentally sick; he shot the president." But it would be awkward to say, "Jones has been mentally sick; he shot the president," or "Jones had been mentally sick; he shot the president." And it would be quite wrong, as well as most odd, to say, "When Jones will be mentally sick, he will shoot the president." (If we thought this about Jones, we would say he is mentally sick.) And it would be odder still to say, "Don't get mentally sick, Jones, you don't want to shoot the president." Humorous as that sounds, the psychiatric and witty dimensions of *mentally sick* would become undistinguishable were we to say, "Jones is mentally sick today; he shoots the president," or "Jones is often mentally sick; he shoots a lot of presidents."

Some of these differences between *sick* and *mentally sick* stem from the fact that we tend to use *sick* to describe states and *mentally sick* to describe characteristics, and that we attribute more permanence to the latter than to the former. Thus, Jones may have pneumonia and may recover from it. Hence, we say, "Jones is sick," and "Jones was sick." But if Jones is an American, so long as Jones is alive, we cannot in the same way say, "Jones is an American," and "Jones was an American" (for the latter means not that he is no longer an American but that he is no longer alive).

The literally or physically *sick*, denoting conditions rather than characteristics, implies no permanency; whereas the metaphorically or mentally *sick*, denoting characteristics rather than conditions, does. It is worth recalling in this connection that permanence has always been the very essence of true madness: when madness was insanity or lunacy, it was incurable; when it became dementia praecox or schizophrenia, it became genetically fixed and had a chronic, downhill course. Even today, *psychotics* can have *remissions* but cannot have *recoveries*.

In the Age of Faith, men and women had to, and wanted to, call their spiritual problems sins and their spiritual authorities fathers, who, in turn, called them children. In the Age of Medicine, men and women have to, and want to, call their spiritual problems sicknesses and their spiritual authorities doctors, who, in turn, call them patients.

The metaphorical character of this sort of language is half-concealed and half-revealed. The words and deeds of men and women reveal that they both know and don't know, want to know and don't want to know, the differences between earth and heaven, man's law and God's law, father and priest, body and mind, medicine and psychiatry, physician and philosopher.

What, it may be asked, is the proper task of science in the face of this sort of situation? Surely, it cannot be to impose its images on those who do not want to see them. But just as surely, it must be to insist that those who want to see them be allowed to do so.

# 12

# Medicine and the State: A *Humanist* Interview

PAUL KURTZ: Dr. Szasz, you have led some vigorous battles on many fronts. What would you say is the key value that you have attempted to defend?

THOMAS SZASZ: If I had to name a single value, it would be individual self-determination or freedom, in a political sense. After all, freedom is an issue only when it is threatened by a person, a group, an organization, or some force. I have tried to identify what the principal forces are that now threaten individual freedom.

KURTZ: And what are they?

SZASZ: In Communist countries, it is the Communist party, the Communist state. In so-called free societies, especially in the United States and England, it is the bureaucratic state, the paternalistic state—or, as I have called it, the therapeutic state. One of the most important aspects or parts of such a state—and hence one of the major threats to individual freedom—is the alliance between medicine and the state, and one particular facet of that alliance, which has concerned me the most, is the acceptance and use of psychiatry as a genuine medical discipline. The alliance is dangerous because it means that the social control of what is really self-determining behavior is called treatment for mental illness and is accepted as something medical rather than moral, as something therapeutic rather than punitive.

KURTZ: How do you think medicine operates in conjunction with the state? Exactly how does it deny freedom?

SZASZ: Let me give you my conclusions about that first, and then we'll fill in the details as we move along. As I see it, medicine does not merely operate in conjunction with the state; in modern industrial societies, medicine is actually a part of the state—it is a sort of *state religion.* I mean that in the sense that most people on both sides of the Iron Curtain now believe in health rather than salvation, in pills rather than prayer, in physicians rather than priests, in medicine and science rather than theology and God. In short, medicine now functions as a state religion much as, for example, Roman Catholicism did in medieval Spain.

KURTZ: You mean that the state and the church are overlapping institutions, not really separate and distinct entities?

SZASZ: Exactly. In Spain, and in other theocratic societies, the state legitimized the church and vice versa. They were intertwined ideologically, economically, politically—in every way. It was an alliance that was very difficult—to say the least—to oppose. That same sort of thing has been happening with medicine and the state in all the civilized countries for the past hundred years or so, especially since the end of the Second World War. The state supports and legitimizes medicine, and medicine in turn supports and legitimizes the state. It's an unholy alliance, if I may put it that way.

KURTZ: Could you illustrate that with an example?

SZASZ: Yes. Medical education is completely controlled by the state—that is, by the state and federal governments. The control is partly economic—much of the money comes from the government; partly educational—the schools have to be approved by state education departments and similar agencies; and partly legal—physicians have to be licensed to practice medicine. And physicians in turn serve the state in both subtle and obvious ways—by reporting births and deaths, controlling deviant behavior, assisting law-enforcement agencies. It goes much further than that, of course. What is health? disease? treatment? The very definition of these things is something that in the last analysis the state determines and medicine accepts and implements. Some examples will show what I mean. Today in New York State, doing an abortion is treatment. Only a year or so ago it was a crime. Locking someone up in a prison called a mental hospital is also considered to be a form of treatment. Why? Because the state says so; the law says so.

KURTZ: Yes, mental hospitalization is a good example.

SZASZ: I have been interested in involuntary mental hospitalization not only because it is such a blatant violation of human rights, but also because it reveals so clearly how we have medicalized certain moral and political problems. If someone wants to do something we really don't like—such as killing himself—then we say he is depressed and lock him up in a mental hospital. How is that possible? Because psychiatry says that depression is a disease; obviously, if you are an American, you should want to live. Look how similar that is to people's being locked up in mental hospitals in the Soviet Union because they criticize the system. Obviously, to the Soviet state and its psychiatrists, anyone who publicly expresses political dissent must be crazy; if he weren't crazy, he would be an obedient Communist.

KURTZ: But in the Soviet Union, that has a political basis—to support the state. Is there the same motive for locking up persons in mental institutions here?

SZASZ: Professor Kurtz, I think we have to come to some agreement about what we mean by political and what we mean by psychiatric. Otherwise, there is a risk that what the Russians do psychiatrically will appear to us as political and what we do will appear to us as psychiatric—and probably vice versa. I would insist that in a fundamental sense all involuntary psychiatry is political. It's the use of the police power of the state against the dissenting citizen. It is as simple as that. What constitutes dissent varies, of course, from country to country. It must. In each case, naturally, dissent is directed against what the citizens don't like, and that differs from country to country.

KURTZ: And people—some people—who deviate from ideological conformity, who dissent in certain socially prohibited ways, may be locked up in psychiatric institutions?

SZASZ: Yes.

KURTZ: What other examples of state control through medicine would support your point? For example, what about drug abuse?

SZASZ: That is a very striking case in point today. Here, again, the state defines—quite arbitrarily from a pharmacological point of view—what is illness and what is treatment, what is permitted and what is prohibited. Taking heroin is addiction. Receiving methadone is treatment. But what's the difference between heroin and methadone? I'll tell you what: it's the same as the difference between Protestantism and Catholicism!

KURTZ: But the public has been told that on heroin you can't function, while on methadone you can; you need methadone to hold down a job, so the methadone-maintenance people argue.

SZASZ: Naturally. How well could you function in post-Reformation Europe if you were a Catholic in a Protestant country, or vice versa? Not very well. So, if you were a Protestant in Paris, it was a good idea to become a Catholic. And if you were a Catholic in London, it was a good idea to become a Protestant. Just so with drugs: it is easier to live in America on methadone than on heroin; the government likes it better that way.

KURTZ: But methadone is a drug. It is administered by the state under certain programs.

SZASZ: Precisely. Methadone is defined as a therapeutic agent and heroin as a dangerous and illegal drug. But heroin itself was developed and first used as a therapeutic agent—as a treatment for morphine addiction. It's sad. But Santayana was so right when he warned that those who cannot remember the past are condemned to repeat it.

KURTZ: So you think in both cases the state merely imposes certain values on the citizens?

SZASZ: Exactly. In the case of religion, certain theological values—for example, you must be a Catholic and not be a Protestant. In the case of medicine, certain therapeutic values—for example, you must take methadone and not heroin.

KURTZ: Is there no difference between these drugs?

SZASZ: Is there no difference between Catholicism and Protestantism?

KURTZ: Yes, but they are also similar.

SZASZ: So are heroin and methadone. They are not identical, but they are similar. And of course it is possible—should the person be otherwise so motivated—to function on both of these drugs, just as it is possible to function as either a Catholic or a Protestant—

provided one is not persecuted for one's religious habit or drug habit! It's the persecution that's disabling, not the drug.

KURTZ: Can you suggest another example to illustrate how the alliance between medicine and the state operates? How it curtails freedom?

SZASZ: Yes, abortion.

KURTZ: The law used to prohibit abortion, but it no longer does, at least in New York State.

SZASZ: Yes, but there are actually two different points to be made here: first, it is the state that determines whether abortion is a crime or a cure; and, second, the state remains intimately involved in abortion even now that it's legal. The state does not simply allow a woman to have an abortion as it allows her to take aspirin. It forces the taxpayer to pay for it. Since abortion is now defined as treatment, if a poor woman has an abortion, the taxpayer pays for it. I think that is a grave moral wrong. After all, an abortion is necessary only because a man and a woman have engaged in sexual intercourse—which may be very nice. It is what's called sumptuary behavior, in fancy language. And so are drinking and smoking. Hence, in my mind, forcing taxpayers to buy abortions for poor women is like forcing taxpayers to buy alcohol or cigarettes for poor men. What mischievous nonsense.

KURTZ: Having the taxpayer pay for abortions, some argue, protects society from unwanted children.

SZASZ: That is a rationalization. It is possible to explain or justify any social policy if one is willing to accept such vague notions as "protection from unwanted children." Lots of children are wanted while they are *in utero* and become unwanted only *in vivo*—after they are born. How about them? Should we kill them to protect society from unwanted children? Actually, the matter of tax-supported abortions raises another interesting issue, one I have never seen mentioned or discussed. I refer to the fact that such abortions actually infringe on the religious liberties of those who, because of their religious convictions, disapprove of abortion—who consider abortion a morally wrongful act. In other words, using the tax monies, say, of devout Catholics to pay for abortions puts the government, however unwittingly, into the business of actively supporting certain kinds of antireligious activities. Now, it may be all right for the ACLU to do that or for any other private group to do that. But if the government does it, it does something that gets uncomfortably close to the sorts of antireligious activities that have characterized Communist societies. The state itself becomes a church; political dogma becomes, in effect, religious dogma, though of course it's never called religion; and we fall into the very trap the First Amendment is supposed to protect us from.

KURTZ: How does your argument affect education and, specifically, medical education?

SZASZ: Let me first make clear that I believe, more or less, in traditional medicine—in so-called Western, scientific medicine. But I do not believe—and this is the cutting edge of my argument—that the state should support only that sort of medical education and should, in effect, outlaw every other kind. It should not, in my opinion, support any kind of medical education. Scientific medicine should compete in the free marketplace of ideas—and in the free economic marketplace—with osteopathy, and homeopathy, and Christian Science, and Zen Buddhism, and what have you.

KURTZ: Would you then have private professional organizations, like the AMA, set standards?

SZASZ: No. I believe the organizations best suited for setting standards are the schools. So there could, and should, be standards in medicine—just as there are in mathematics or religion, but those standards are neither set nor enforced by the state. I have come to believe that if we value personal freedom and dignity, we must be satisfied with nothing less than a complete separation between medicine and the state—a separation analogous to that between church and state guaranteed in the First Amendment.

KURTZ: But health and welfare are basic points in the Constitution.

SZASZ: But how could health be more important to the general welfare than religion? Not to mention the vexing questions of what is health, and what is religion, and again, who has the final authority to define them. The classic American answer to this dilemma was that the way to promote true religion (not *the* true religion) was by promoting religious freedom and by opposing the establishment of a state religion—of religious monopoly, as it were. The basic concept of American political liberty is thus rooted in the idea that since the established churches used to threaten pluralism, diversity, and personal freedom, the state should guarantee the impossibility of any church's using the power of the state to impose its views on anybody who does not want them imposed on him. That is the essential problem we now face with respect to medicine. So my view does not imply that every form of medical practice is as good as any other, any more than defending religious tolerance implies that one thinks any system of religious beliefs and practices is as good as any other.

KURTZ: Then you think that medicine is a kind of religion and ought to be pluralistic without the state's determining one point of view against another.

SZASZ: Determining and *imposing* that point of view!

KURTZ: Would there then be professional bodies? Would there be any norms or standards of correct practice and therapy?

SZASZ: Of course, there could be and would be, just as there are in other professions today, such as mathematics. If IBM wants to hire a mathematician, it can't look to the state to tell it who is qualified. But it can find out if the man has a Ph.D. from Harvard or MIT. Or the company can set its own standards, can make its own assessment of the applicant's capabilities.

KURTZ: Your point, then, is that the state should not license doctors.

SZASZ: Certainly not. The licensing of doctors is the *symbol* of what I am talking about. It's as if the state would license Catholic priests for the ministry—and would prohibit all other clergymen to practice religion because they are quacks.

KURTZ: But then who should do the licensing?

SZASZ: There should be *no* licensing.

KURTZ: No licensing? Anyone could practice medicine?

SZASZ: Of course.

KURTZ: But how would you protect the public? What about the quacks?

SZASZ: Professor Kurtz, the idea that licensing doctors protects the public is one of the most uncritically accepted falsehoods of our day.

KURTZ: What do you mean?

SZASZ: Well, suppose a professor of medicine or surgery at the University of London were to come to New York; could he practice medicine? Or suppose a professor of medicine or surgery at Harvard—or the State University of New York—were to move to Miami because it's warmer there; could he practice there?

KURTZ: No, not without first passing the state medical-board examinations.

SZASZ: Exactly. And that is to protect the public? Hardly. I grant, of course, that licensure examinations may, *inter alia,* also protect the public. But I insist that their first and foremost function is to protect physicians, the medical profession, from too much competition. In short, medical licensure is a method for preserving a closed union shop for physicians—for maintaining an artificial shortage of doctors. And the whole thing has been successfully palmed off on the American public as something done for its protection.

KURTZ: So how should the public be protected? Doesn't it need protection from incompetent medical practitioners?

SZASZ: Oh, I agree that people need protection—but not only from bad, stupid, inept, greedy, evil doctors; they need protection also from bad parents and children, husbands and wives, mothers-in-law, bureaucrats, teachers, politicians—the list is endless. And then of course, they'll need protection from the protectors! So the question of how people should be protected from incompetent medical practitioners is really a part of the larger question of how they should be protected from the countless hazards of life. That is a vastly complicated problem for which there are no simple solutions. The first line of protection for the public lies, I would say, in self-protection. People must grow up and learn to protect themselves—or suffer the consequences. There can be no freedom without risk and responsibility. More specifically, the public could look to what school the doctor graduated from and could set up all sorts of unofficial testing mechanisms—sort of consumers' bureaus. The possibilities of nongovernmental checks on competence are immense. The trouble is no one is interested in even thinking along those lines nowadays.

KURTZ: Many people know very little about medicine. They may go to a man who claims to know what he is doing but doesn't.

SZASZ: That's true. But what I am talking about now is a long-range view. It's a view that couldn't be implemented overnight. To make it meaningful, practical, we would have to envision corresponding changes in education, in people's interest in, and knowledge about, their own bodies, about drugs, and so forth.

KURTZ: Why do you think that people don't know more about medicine?

SZASZ: There are many reasons. One is because they aren't taught anything about it. You know, most professions thrive on mystification, on keeping the public in the dark—despite all the protestations about popularizing medical knowledge. I have always thought that twelve-year-olds and thirteen-year-olds could be taught a great deal about how the body works—really works; it's no more difficult either to teach or to learn that than is algebra or French grammar.

KURTZ: You would teach medicine in high school?

SZASZ: Certainly. Not how to take out an appendix, but how the body works, what doctors do—the basic principles and facts of phsysiology, pharmacology, the major diseases that affect man and the treatments for them. Real information—what's in medical textbooks—not the lies children are now taught in the name of sex education, drug education, health education. None of that is possible, however, so long as education is a state monopoly.

KURTZ: Why not?

SZASZ: Because the doctor is a priest who teaches only his religion, and only to a select few. As a priest protected by the state, the doctor becomes the keeper of all kinds of secrets. Remember the Latin prescriptions and the diagnostic mumbo jumbo to keep from patients the knowledge of what ails them. Even today, physicians seriously contemplate when patients should and should not be told they have cancer. The whole thing is really quite absurd once one stands back and looks at it as an anthropologist might at another culture. Magic used to be used as medicine. Now medicine is used as magic.

KURTZ: But that is not all the doctors' fault?

SZASZ: Certainly not. I wouldn't want to give the impression that I think it is. It takes two to tango. Freud was quite right in emphasizing that one of the greatest passions men have is the passion *not* to know—to repress, to mystify—the obvious. Thus, there is a sort of conspiracy between people who do not want to know, who want to remain stupid, and experts who will lie to them, who will make a profession out of stupefying them. The priests used to do a good job of that. Now the physicians do it. And, above all, the politicians are in there pitching to make sure people hear all the lies they want to hear.

KURTZ: I think much of it comes from our religious prohibitions.

SZASZ: Only in a historical sense, not otherwise. It's easy to blame religion where I think we should blame, if blame we must, human nature. Religion—formal religion—is not very important in those areas anymore. How could it be when Blue Cross now pays for abortions? And yet, in New York State, a woman cannot buy a diaphragm in a drugstore even if she knows her size. She must have a prescription for it from a physician. I mention that again to note its symbolic significance: it reveals the ceremonial, magical role and power of the doctor.

KURTZ: Can we go back to heroin and methadone to focus and highlight your position? What is your position on so-called dangerous drugs? Should there be no controls?

SZASZ: None for adults. I don't see how anyone can take seriously the idea of personal self-determination and responsibility and not insist on his right to take anything he wants to take. The American government simply does not have the right to tell him what he may or may not take—any more than it has the right to tell him what he may or may not think. That doesn't mean, obviously, that it's a good thing to take certain drugs. It most assuredly can be a very bad thing. But a person must, if he is to be free, have the right to poison and kill himself. As, indeed, he now does with tobacco, but not with marijuana; with alcohol, but not with heroin.

KURTZ: You agree, obviously, with John Stuart Mill's *On Liberty*, which argues the same way.

SZASZ: Yes. Mill taught us all this. We really have no choice in the matter—that is, of drugs and self-injury and suicide; we must either agree with him or commit ourselves to a sort of unlimited inconsistency and hypocrisy.

KURTZ: Why can't we have a balance between personal freedom and state protection?

SZASZ: We can in some areas but not in others. For example, we can have state protection with respect to genuine public-health issues, such as sewage disposal or water purification. But we can't if we try to go beyond that and expect the state to provide us with a sort of metaphorical public health—for example, by putting things into water or bread that are supposedly good for us. There are things the state can't do and shouldn't try to do. I refer to the libertarian principle that the state shouldn't do what the people can do for themselves. The state can't protect people beyond a certain, very minimal, point without denying them their freedom of choice. When it tries, the result is a disaster—or, to be precise, two kinds of disasters. In the free world, the state's ostensible efforts to protect the people from medical harm have gone hand in hand with the most blatant state-supported programs of "poisoning" people—for example, the opium wars in the nineteenth century (which were waged to spread the use of opium, not to curtail it) or the agricultural supports to tobacco growers today and the use of federal funds to encourage cigarette smoking abroad. In the totalitarian countries, the cost of trying to achieve a balance between personal freedom and state protection has been even higher: there it has required the liquidation of the most elementary human rights, such as the right to property, to a free press—even the right to leave one's country.

KURTZ: Well, are you against laws for prescriptions?

SZASZ: Of course.

KURTZ: There should be no laws . . .

SZASZ: There should be no *prescriptions!*

KURTZ: But suppose my wife had a cold. She likes to take antibiotics, and I worry about it—about whether they are necessary, whether she may develop a sensitivity to them, that sort of thing. How would you protect the public against that?

SZASZ: I am looking to protection through self-control. Today, without prescriptions, people can buy lye and all sorts of very dangerous cleaning fluids, and they know quite well how to protect themselves from those things. Really, amazingly well. Where there is a will, there is a way. But where there is no will—well, then, I would let the individual suffer the consequences rather than punish the whole society by prohibiting the "abused" substance.

KURTZ: You feel it's really impossible to protect people from themselves?

SZASZ: Impossible as well as immoral, in a sense. The problem we touch on here is really as old as mankind. It goes to the very roots of freedom and responsibility—and humanism—to the roots of the question of what is man. It's all contained in the parable of the Fall. Who was the first pusher? The serpent. And who were the first addicts? Eve and Adam. And what was the consequence of that "original addiction"? Freedom! It's all there, in the first few pages of the Old Testament. But who reads that nowadays? And who reads it with open eyes or with an open mind?

KURTZ: Many people agree with some of that, or with much of it, but then they say, "What about children?" Would you let children buy any drug they want?

SZASZ: No, I would not. In a practical sense, for the present, I think the method we have developed with respect to alcohol is quite sensible: children can't buy it, but if they use it, say, at home, it's none of the law's business. So a twelve-year-old can't go into a liquor store and buy a bottle of gin. And that law is well enforced, as far as I know. The point is that the control of children—what children do with respect to drugs—is, and should be, a problem for the child's parents and, as the child grows older, for the child himself. We have forgotten the simple fact that childhood is the period of life when one should learn self-control—and if one doesn't, then one will be an adult lacking self-control.

KURTZ: But how do you deal with those cases where you have a breakdown of the family, where there is increasing lack of responsibility among parents?

SZASZ: I don't know how to deal with such cases. I only know how *not* to deal with them. I know that the breakdown of the family cannot and should not be dealt with by treating the whole society as a child. But that is just what we do now: because some children are not controlled by their parents and misbehave as a result, we treat all adults as if they were misbehaving children. The result is the paternalistic state—the therapeutic state, as I have called it—that we now have.

KURTZ: Dr. Szasz, you emphasize that the alliance between medicine and the state, between psychiatry and the state, is similar to the alliance between religion and the state. Do you find that in other fields as well—for example, in the law?

SZASZ: Certainly, the problem is not limited to medicine or psychiatry. In totalitarian countries, where the whole legal profession is an arm of the state, really a servant of the state, we have something quite similar to what is developing in Western countries with respect to the medical profession. However, in American law, the situation is not quite so bad. We have a strong, viable tradition that articulates and legitimizes a dual role for the criminal law: on the one hand, the law serves the state to protect it from the citizen; on the other hand, it serves the citizen to protect him from the state. And in civil law, of course, the law serves to protect the citizens from one another. Thus, there is a general understanding—a popular appreciation—that lawyers and courts deal with conflicts and that in conflicts both parties are entitled to representation. We have nothing like that in medicine, and that is just the problem.

KURTZ: You think we need a bill of rights for patients?

SZASZ: No, I don't think that would do it. I think that would be just a piece of paper. There has to be a popular understanding first—a common-sense appreciation of the difference between illness as a biological and medical concept and conflict as a personal and political concept.

KURTZ: Why is there this confusion, this misunderstanding?

SZASZ: There are good reasons for it. In medicine, the traditional image of the problem is that of a patient fighting against his disease; in that situation, the disease—the infection, cancer, what not—is the adversary and the doctor the ally. This then is the basis of the misunderstanding for all the medical situations in which this imagery, this explanation, doesn't apply—in which the physician is the patient's adversary, not his ally. For example, in what we now call drug addiction, the drug is the ally and the doctor is the adversary; also, in what we now call serious mental illness, I would say the psychosis—the delusion—is the ally and again the doctor is the adversary. But medicine and the law do not recognize that, and people do not recognize it either—except when they are the victims, and then it's usually too late.

KURTZ: So what is the answer? What would help if not a bill of rights for patients?

SZASZ: I think a conceptual and economic separation between medicine and the state must come first, and of course civil libertarians and others—philosophers, writers, sociologists—could help to separate those medical situations where the physician is the patient's ally from those where he is his adversary.

KURTZ: Now, are there other institutions in society that also undermine freedom—since to you freedom is apparently the most important value? We talked about medicine and the law; what about education?

SZASZ: Well, many of the things I have said about medicine others have said about education, and I quite agree with them—Paul Goodman, for example, and Bertrand Russell before him. To the extent that education is financed and legitimized by the state, education becomes propaganda. That problem is even larger and older than that of medicine. How is the independence and integrity of the educator maintained? What is taught and to whom? One has to think only of Socrates to realize how ancient the problem is.

KURTZ: In modern society, still another problem is the development of large institutions and organizations independent of the state. Many people now consider that large corporations, industrial firms, function like states and that they too can jeopardize freedom, can encroach on individual liberty. What would be your view on that?

SZASZ: My view is—and it is certainly not a very original view—that any organization, any institution, public or private—the state, the church, a profession, a business—tends to become repressive as it grows beyond a certain size. Of course, it may even start out to be repressive; repression may be its very *raison d'être*. But even if it is not that at the outset, repression soon becomes one of its goals, one of its interests. That is because as soon as any organization or institution becomes established, it will come in conflict with other organizations or institutions with competing interests. The larger and more successful group will try not only to promote its interests, products, markets, and so forth, but also to suppress and to annihilate its competitors. In that sense, any group, any organization, is by its very nature repressive. That is an idea that goes back, of course, to Montesquieu and the Founding Fathers. It is the reason why libertarians have always insisted that anyone who values the individual and his freedom must oppose the accumulation of monolithic power regardless of who accumulates it and for what purpose. Power accumulated for good reasons—for doing good—is the most dangerous of all. Who can be against good health today?

Who could be against good religion in the past? Who can be against good education? After all, we know that two and two makes four. Why should anyone be allowed to say they make five? Because if we prevent people from teaching that, we unleash a complex process that leads inevitably to the accumulation of monopolistic educational power with all its dreadful consequences.

KURTZ: Many people look, however, to the state as a countervailing power. They regard private corporations and organizations as systems of power that impose their will on the individual, and they believe that the state functions as the protector of the individual. For example, the state sets standards in medicine, in education. And we have antitrust laws, the Federal Trade Commission, the Federal Communications Commission. Are you unsympathetic to all that?

SZASZ: The American state has become an exceedingly complicated social instrument. Parts of it do protect the individual, and other parts of it injure the individual. Now, of course, the state does have other functions than the protection of individual freedom, and I accept that. For that very reason, however, I think it's foolish to trust the state very far for what it does for the individual. It usually does more *to* him than *for* him.

KURTZ: Now, as a libertarian, would you be opposed to socialism? I mean could one combine libertarianism and socialism?

SZASZ: Well, before I answer that, could you say just what you mean by socialism?

KURTZ: Socialism is being redefined today. I mean simply the idea that the state owns some of the basic means of production; perhaps also that the state would enter more and more into producing goods and providing services that are not produced in the private sector, and that it would be concerned with social welfare. That is true, for example, of British socialism.

SZASZ: If that is what you mean, then I would say not only that socialism is incompatible with libertarianism but that it is one of its most dangerous and powerful enemies. I am not an anarchist, though, as you know, that ideology exercises a certain charm for many libertarians. I consider anarchism unrealistic, impractical. Man is a social being. We can live only in groups; we must live in groups; we must have certain kinds of social cooperation. We now secure such cooperation in part through what we call the state. But I believe with traditional libertarians that the state should do as little as possible in competition with individual initiative. The state should provide for national defense and exercise the police function and some types of regulatory functions. But the more the state does beyond those things, the more it becomes an enemy of the people. The best examples of that at present are state-supplied education and state-supplied medicine. Look at our *public* schools. Look at our *state* hospitals. Who wants them? Not the consumers "committed" to them! Those are the two roads to totalitarianism. In Communism, all that is done overtly, of course. There the state controls everything. In the so-called free societies, we move toward similar controls by letting the state control education and medicine.

KURTZ: There are differences though.

SZASZ: Of course there are. But the trend, the direction, is toward state control. And the end result tends to be the same—the reduction of individual choice.

KURTZ: Dr. Szasz, you noted the collectivist-totalitarian trends in Western societies, trends emanating from the state control of education and medicine. What about the difference between the Communist societies and the free ones?

SZASZ: Do you know where I think one of the most important practical social differences lies between the Communist and non-Communist societies? In the fourth estate.

KURTZ: The newspapers?

SZASZ: Yes, the free press. I think it's astonishing—and wonderfully revealing—how people defend the freedom of the press while they do not defend nearly so much, or not at all, freedom of education or freedom of medicine. We think it's absolutely essential that the press be free—that the newspapers be able to print what they want—and that Americans should have the right to read what they want. But we do not think they should have the right to buy penicillin without a doctor's prescription. Why can't you buy penicillin? Because it can hurt you? Can't lies hurt you? The newspapers are full of lies. The magazines are full of lies. Why doesn't the government protect people from lies? Because that would be a violation of the First Amendment. And that's fine. But there is a chink in the First Amendment, and that chink is called health and medicine and treatment. Anything that can be brought under that umbrella—that can be so classified—can be manipulated and regulated and prohibited by the government. Just one quick example: tobacco, which is a plant, is classified as an agricultural product and is promoted by the government; marijuana, which is another plant, is classified as a dangerous drug and is prohibited by the government.

KURTZ: Is it a matter of degree, as to personal freedom, between the totalitarian countries and the Western democracies?

SZASZ: That's complicated. In part, it's a matter of degree; in part, it's a matter of law; in part, it's a matter of economic arrangements. And perhaps most of all, it's a matter of tradition. After all, I believe—and again I draw on a long list of other opinions here—that in the West there is a significant tradition concerning the value of the individual—a strong feeling for individual liberty; there is no comparable tradition or feeling in the East.

KURTZ: In your view, then, humanism draws deeply from the well of freedom—freedom of the individual—and considers it to be its central value.

SZASZ: Yes. That would be my view of humanism. But obviously there are other views, other definitions. I need hardly tell you that. I might mention here, in conclusion, that there seem to me really two entirely different ways of approaching what humanism is—of identifying it. One is by trying to define the good life, the good person—tolerance, openness, love, reason, whatever the definer values. The articulation and realization of that kind of life—that life-style, to use a current cliché—then becomes humanism. The other approach is not to give it such a psychological or moral definition at all. It is to say instead—and this is the view I prefer—that humanism is the result, the consequence, of an optimal or maximal kind of pluralism and diversity in society. In that sense, humanism is not this or that way of living, but the diversity that results from the economic, political, and psychological circumstances that permit one person to live one way and another, another way.

KURTZ: So humanism would maximize the autonomy of the individual to choose as he sees fit.

SZASZ: Exactly. And such autonomy has no meaning outside of a political and socioeconomic context that provides and protects the range of choices available.

KURTZ: So it's not only freedom for the individual but a free society. They go hand in hand.

SZASZ: Yes. But I would prefer to reassert the political dimension of everything that we have been talking about. Humanism is usually thought of primarily in ethical and psychological terms. I want to emphasize the political criteria and ideas. And among those, there is one notion I want to single out, and that is *dissent*. After all, authorities never object to people agreeing with them. But they get unhappy and often quite nasty when people disagree with them. So it's disagreement that must be nurtured and protected. In short, instead of thinking of humanism as this or that kind of life-style or ideology, I think we should think of it more as the right to disagree and reject authority—religious authority, educational authority, medical authority—and of course the right to take one's chances with one's own judgment and decision. That would be a definition of humanism in terms of dissent rather than in terms of affirmation. Of course, we could view that as the affirmation of the individual against the group, of the layman against the expert. It's a simple idea, but still full of unexplored promises and possibilities. The idea is this: the Fall was really not a fall but a rise—a rise from infantilism to humanism.

It is error alone which needs the support of government. Truth can stand by itself. . . . The way to silence religious disputes, is to take no notice of them. Let us too give this experiment fair play, and get rid, while we may, of those tyrannical laws. It is true, we are yet secured against them by the spirit of the times. I doubt whether the people of this country would suffer an execution of heresy, or three years' imprisonment for not comprehending the mysteries of the Trinity. But is that spirit of the people an infallible, a permanent reliance? Is it government? Besides, the spirit of the times may alter, will alter. Our rulers will become corrupt, our people careless. . . . From the conclusion of this war we shall be going down hill. It will not then be necessary to resort every moment to the people for support. They will be forgotten, therefore, and their rights disregarded. They will forget themselves, but in the sole faculty of making money, and will never think of uniting to effect a due respect for their rights.

Thomas Jefferson, "Notes on the State of Virginia" (1781)

# Index